Approaches to Teaching Health Care in Social Work

A Compendium of Model Syllabi

Compiled by

Valire Carr Copeland, Vivian Jackson,
Lily Jarman-Rohde, Anita L. Rosen,
and Glenn Stone

In conjunction with the Council on Social Work Education's

Commission on Social Work Practice

From the Council on Social Work Education's Series

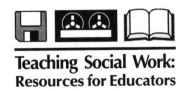

Teaching Social Work:
Resources for Educators

Council on Social Work Education
1600 Duke Street, Suite 300
Alexandria, VA 22314-3421

Printed in the United States of America

Approaches to Teaching Health Care in Social Work: A Compendium of Model Syllabi

Compiled by Valire Carr Copeland, Vivian Jackson, Lily Jarman-Rohde, Anita L. Rosen, and Glenn Stone

ISBN 0-87293-068-8

❖ Table of Contents ❖

❖ Preface ❖

Social work in health care is a fluid and dynamic area of practice that has been undergoing tremendous change over the past five years. Among the recent changes and challenges are: managed care, developments in medical technology and pharmaceuticals that increase life expectancy, rising consumer expectations about quality of life and quality of care, changing professional roles and locus of service, new case management arrangements, and the recognition of the importance of mental health in physical well-being. In an effort to assist undergraduate and graduate social work programs to prepare students for the demands of practice in today's health care environment, the Commission on Social Work Practice of the Council on Social Work Education (CSWE) presents this collection of course syllabi.

The course outlines chosen were selected from the response to a CSWE call for submissions. The Practice commission's review committee used the CSWE Instrument for Evaluating Course Outlines, included in the Appendix, as well as several other criteria for selection. We sought outlines that were representative of both BSW and MSW programs and courses that reflected a spectrum of social work curriculum content. Included are courses in policy, practice, human behavior, and research, as well as courses in "Special Topics" and advanced practice, those from a concentration area curriculum, generalist courses, and integrative courses.

Other review criteria included an interest in a lifespan approach to health and social work, a strengths perspective to intervention, and recognition of the interaction of health with mental health. We sought content on values and ethics, death and dying, diversity and health, and biopsychosocial aspects of illness. The review committee also had particular interest in the interdisciplinary nature of social work in health practice, which was reflected in the fact that several of the courses were cross-listed with other departments, were taught by interdisciplinary faculty, or made use of guest lecturers from a variety of settings.

The rapidly changing context of providing health care in this society makes it critical that those who teach social work health courses are able to change and adapt content to remain current and relevant. The courses in this compendium are successful examples of this endeavor. In addition to the currency of content, these course syllabi are able to balance a mixture of seminal works on health care with more current books, articles, and other material on the subject.

In reviewing the syllabi for the project, several themes emerged. First among them was the inclusion of content on special populations within the syllabi. The selected syllabi covered content on such special populations as women, minorities of color, gay men and lesbians, the poor, and individuals with mental and physical disabilities.

Another theme that emerged was the emphasis on "current" health topics. Various syllabi included content on: managed care, long-term care, health care for the aging population, women's health issues, maternal and child health, interdisciplinary collaboration and teamwork, family-centered care, cognitive factors in health and illness, HIV/AIDS, the genetic basis of health, illness prevention and health promotion, case management, cultural issues, community-based care, continuum-of-care issues, employee assistance programs, and more.

The included syllabi not only cover a variety of content and issues, but also offer a variety of readings, course assignments, and teaching methodologies. Examples noted in this area include: (a) use of real-world examples and assignments, (b) use of technology, (c) ethnographic interviews and personal research, (d) personal journals and logs, and (e) student presentations.

The syllabi also present a variety of methods of instruction including: (a) use of guest lecturers; (b) field trips; (c) use of websites, course home pages, bulletin boards, discussion groups, and e-mail; and (d) interdisciplinary team teaching. Of course, more traditional forms of presentations were included as well (i.e., lecture, video, discussion), but these courses help remind us that part of effective teaching is finding new and creative ways to involve students in the learning process. The use of technology in the classroom is an excellent example of how social work educators can help prepare students for the expectations regarding technological know-how that they will undoubtedly encounter once they are in the work force.

Future Needs

This collection of course outlines is a first step to better prepare social workers for health care practice. Given the rapidly changing nature of such practice, no collection will provide all the "answers" about what to teach. Nevertheless, these outlines do provide content, methods, and resources that convey current conceptions of preparing and challenging students to practice in a dynamic, complex, and fragmented health care system.

This sampling of curricula does not allow the reader to assess other courses in various programs or to predict whether students are able to grasp the biopsychosocial needs of diverse populations in hospitals, nursing homes, hospices, rehabilitation facilities, and home- and community-based settings. The diversity of populations, the changing role of health care workers, and the variety of health care settings and conditions facing the social worker all present an array of professional issues that demand creativity, currency, and substance. We hope that this sample of exemplary syllabi will serve as a catalyst to the development of future curricula that will sustain a vital role for professional social workers in a changing health care environment.

A number of people were instrumental in making this collection possible. We want to thank CSWE for its interest and support of the Commission on Social Work Practice, and we want to commend the Practice commission and its chair, Dan Weisman of Rhode Island College, for encouraging us. Special thanks to Lily Jarman-Rohde of the University of Michigan for writing a successful proposal for this project, and to commission members Valire Carr Copeland (University of Pittsburgh) and Vivian Jackson (Child Welfare Advisor to the Washington Business Group on Health) for their excellent work as expert reviewers.

Glenn Stone
Assistant Professor, Department of Family Studies and Social Work
Miami University

Anita Rosen
Project Coordinator, Preparing Gerontology-Competent Social Workers
Council on Social Work Education

❖ Foreword ❖

In the interest of improving the availability and quality of instructional materials in social work, the Council on Social Work Education's Publications and Media Commission has developed a series entitled *Teaching Social Work: Resources for Educators*. This collection of course outlines on social work in health care, compiled by Glenn Stone and Anita Rosen, in conjunction with the Council's Commission on Social Work Practice, represents a component of this effort.

Although the syllabi in this collection are not intended to serve as official, CSWE-approved models for curriculum development, they are examples of high-quality, peer-reviewed resources that may be of use to social work faculty at a variety of institutions.

Ann Weick
Chair, Publications and Media Commission

University of Maryland–Baltimore County
Department of Social Work
Baltimore, MD

Course Title: Case Management with Vulnerable Populations (SOWK 390P)
Spring 1998

Course Instructor: Betsy Vourlekis

COURSE DESCRIPTION

This social work elective provides an in-depth examination of a service modality and growing arena of professional practice that is a prominent feature of human service delivery systems meeting a wide range of individual and family needs. While the current proliferation of case management stems from the intersecting realities of service fragmentation, cost containment pressures, and privatization that characterize the American welfare system, the essential case management focus of person-in-situation has long been the concern of social work direct practice. Nevertheless, case management today is characterized by a number of different models, and is considered to be in the professional practice domain of a number of professions in addition to social work.

This course focuses on one model, namely, direct service, interactive case management programs, and the case manager as a service provider within these programs. In programs as diverse as child or adult protective services, hospital-based discharge planning, community support for persons with serious mental illness, care coordination for persons with AIDS, and services to the elderly—to name just a few—the goal of this case management model is to coordinate, integrate, or manage an array of resources and services that effectively and efficiently address the situations of people who have complex, long-term needs.

Often described as boundary-spanning practice, social work case management requires simultaneous involvement with a client (plus client's family/significant others) as well as other helpers and resource systems. All phases of the problem-solving process, from relationship building to evaluation and termination, necessarily focus on both client and service system levels. Concepts from ecosystems, social network, and cognitive-behavioral theory will guide understanding of the case manager's field of interest, and the dynamics of both obstacles and opportunities for change within a case management situation.

Students will choose an application of the case management model in a specific field of health/human service, or specific target population. Using this application as the unit of attention, students will examine (1) specific policy initiatives that support case management; (2) the biopsychosocial circumstances and special issues of individuals and their significant others who are the target group; (3) nine generic case management functions in a problem-solving process; (4) specific skills and strategies for working with both individuals and service systems in implementing the nine core functions; and (5) ethical concerns. As a result of this critical analysis, students will come to recognize that ambitious and, at times, conflicting expectations routinely confront the case manager. Consequently they also will explore common sources of frustration and worker burnout, as well as examine empirical evidence concerning the actual effectiveness of case management programs.

The course will build from and apply students' basic understanding of (1) specific policies and programs by fields of practice, developed in SOWK 260; and (2) complex life-spaces consisting of multiple, interacting biological, psychological, and social systems, developed in SOWK 388. Basic familiarity with the social work helping process and interpersonal skills is assumed.

LEARNING OBJECTIVES

Knowledge Objectives

1. To understand the historical and current policy context that shapes case management practice.
2. To understand the key differences among prominent models of case management, and the distinguishing features of social work case management practice.
3. To understand the generic process and functions of social work case management regardless of setting or client population.
4. To understand the complex biopsychosocial needs and circumstances of vulnerable individuals and their families who are the recipients of case management services.
5. To understand the complex service system expectations and circumstances that shape case management practice.

Skill Objectives

1. To use systematic information gathering (including research literature) to enhance understanding of client life space and needs and the policy context of case management practice.
2. To apply theoretical concepts that promote a system-spanning view of a case management situation and the dynamic interactions within it.
3. To recognize and analyze the process and functions of case management in a specific application.
4. To recognize and design specific helping strategies at both the client and service system levels and at each stage of the helping process that further case management objectives.
5. To use self-reflection in considering the multiple demands of the case manager role.

Attitude Objectives

1. To commit to the exercise of social work values in practicing social work case management.
2. To develop a balanced stance with respect to the dual accountability to client and service system in the case manager role.
3. To develop increased comfort with ethical dilemmas that arise in the course of practice, and with a process to resolve them.
4. To maintain a constructive and professionally respectful stance toward other helpers and systems even in the face of obstacles and conflicts.
5. To build confidence in one's own potential as a case manager, while recognizing the legitimate expertise of other professionals who also claim the role.

OUTCOME COMPETENCIES

In addition to demonstrating intellectual mastery of the knowledge and skills outlined above, successful completion of this course means that the student has demonstrated the following practice competencies:

1. Can recognize the processes of the social work generic problem-solving approach in actual case management practice.

2. Can identify and analyze the impact of salient policy directives and the community and organizational context that shape case management practice.

3. Can design an appropriate strategy to address an obstacle to the case management process at both the individual client system level and at the service system level.

4. Can communicate at an acceptable professional level both verbally and in writing.

5. Can accept feedback from colleagues concerning one's professional thinking and behavior; can provide constructive feedback to colleagues on same.

6. Is accountable and dependable in meeting professional obligations engendered by the course.

REQUIRED TEXT

Vourlekis, B. S., & Greene, R. R. (1992). *Social Work Case Management*. New York: Aldine de Gruyter.

COURSE REQUIREMENTS AND GRADING

This upper-level social work elective will be conducted as a seminar, assuming active participation in a number of different ways by each participant: (1) attendance at class sessions is assumed and will be considered in your final grade; (2) discussion based on ideas and information from assigned readings will be a part of each class session, so required reading must be completed on a regular basis; (3) peer consultation, sharing of experiences, participation in and constructive critique of class role-plays, and serving as a resource consultant or resource investigator are all expected activities for class participation.

There is one major paper for the course and four "pop" or unscheduled quizzes. Quizzes will be based on the required reading for each week. The final paper will be a Case Management Analysis Portfolio consisting of four sections. Please see the separate guidelines and instructions for this assignment.

The weighting of these components in computing your final grade is as follows:

Written Case Management Analysis Portfolio	45 points
Best three out of four quiz scores	35 points
Attendance and participation in class	20 points

COURSE OUTLINE

UNIT I: History and Policy Context of Case Management

In this unit you will learn about

- Why case management means different things in different programs.
- How case management came to be necessary in human service delivery.
- Policies that define what case management is.
- The settings and vulnerable client populations for which case management approaches are typically used.
- Needs and beliefs of vulnerable clients.

Required Reading

1. Vourlekis & Greene, Chapter 1, "The Policy and Professional Context of Case Management Practice"

2. Rose, S. M., & Moore, V. L. (1995). "Case Management." In R. L. Edwards (Ed.-in-Chief), *Encyclopedia of Social Work* (19th ed.), pp. 335-339. Washington, DC: NASW Press.

3. Rothman, J. (1994). "The Severely Vulnerable: An Emergent Clientele and Practice Mode." In J. Rothman, *Practice with Highly Vulnerable Clients*, pp. 3-15. Englewood Cliffs, NJ: Prentice Hall.

4. Gary, L. (1987). Attitudes of black adults toward community mental health centers. *Hospital and Community Psychiatry, 38*, 1100-1105.

5. Applewhite, S. L. (1995). Curanderismo: Demystifying the health beliefs and practices of elderly Mexican Americans. *Health and Social Work, 20*, 247-253.

UNIT II: Social Work Case Management as Boundary-Spanning Practice

In this unit you will learn about

- Who does case management and what difference it makes.
- What the dual focus of social work case management is.
- Using an ecosystems framework to clarify individual, family, community, and organizational influences in case management.
- How social work values influence case management practice.

Required Reading

1. Vourlekis & Greene, Chapter 2
2. O'Connor, G. (1988). Case management: System and practice. *Social Casework, 69*, 97-106.
3. Perloff, J. (1996). Medicaid managed care and urban poor people. *Health and Social Work, 21*, 189-195.

UNIT III: The Functions and Process of Social Work Case Management

In this unit you will learn about

- Eight generic functions of the social work case manager.
- How program and agency purpose and role within the service delivery system influence functions.
- How clients' needs influence functions.
- How staffing and resources influence functions.
- Assessing needs and resources from the client's perspective.
- Cultural competence and case management functions.

Required Reading

1. Vourlekis & Greene, Chapters 3, 4, 6, 7, and 10
2. *NASW Standards for Social Work Case Management* (handout in class)
3. Rothman, J. (1991). A model of case management: Toward empirically based practice. *Social Work, 36*, 520-528.
4. Dill, A. (1993). Defining needs, defining systems: A critical analysis. *The Gerontologist, 33*, 453-460.

UNIT IV: Skills and Strategies at the Client and Service System Levels

In this unit you will learn about

- Key skills for each of the eight case management functions.
- Characteristic obstacles and problems at both the client system and service system levels.
- Social network intervention strategies (building new ties, maintaining existing ties, and enhancing family ties).
- Case and cause advocacy.
- Dealing with bias and oppression in service systems.
- Issues in collaborative practice.

Required Reading

1. Vourlekis & Greene, Chapters 8, 9, and 13
2. Singleton-Bowie, S. (1995). The effect of mental health practitioners' racial sensitivity on African-Americans' perception of service. *Social Work Research, 19,* 238-244.
3. Biegel, D. E, Tracy, E. M., & Corvo, K. (1994) Strengthening social networks. *Health and Social Work, 19,* 206-216.
4. Kadushin, G. (1996). Gay men with AIDS and their families of origin. *Health and Social Work, 21,* 141-149.
5. Germain, C. (1984) Collaborative practice in health care: The social work function. In C. Germain, *Social Work Practice in Health Care* (chp. 8, pp. 198-229). New York: Free Press.
6. Mizrahi, T., & Abramson, J. (1985). Sources of strain between physicians and social workers: Implications for social workers in health care settings. *Social Work in Health Care, 10,* 33-51.

UNIT V: Ethics, Accountability, and the Affective Demands of Case Management

In this unit you will learn about
- Steps to thinking through ethical dilemmas and conflicts.
- Common approaches to showing results and demonstrating problems with systems.
- Recognizing common signs of worker burnout and strategies to deal with them.

Required Reading

1. Vourlekis & Greene, Chapter 12
2. Kane, R. A. (1988). Case management: Ethical pitfalls on the road to high-quality managed care. *QRB [Quality Review Bulletin], 14,* 161-166.
3. Gambrill, E. (1997). Maintaining skills and staying happy in your work. In *Social Work Practice: A Critical Thinker's Guide,* pp. 617-624. New York: Oxford University Press,
4. Nelson, J. L. (1992). Taking families seriously. *Hastings Center Report, 4,* 6-12.

APPENDIX

CASE MANAGEMENT ANALYSIS PORTFOLIO

This is a written assignment consisting of 4 parts. Parts I and II are due the first class after spring break, and will be graded and returned to you. Parts III and IV are due at the last class. At that time you will hand in all four parts, along with a bibliography, so that your entire portfolio can be evaluated for a grade.

Your portfolio will consist of your research, analysis, and application of course material to case management practice in a specific field of health/human services, or specific target population. Early in the course you will select your focus from a list I will provide. Complete all four parts of the portfolio using the same field/population. Additional guidelines concerning each part of the portfolio will be distributed as the class progresses.

Part I: Policy background

Locate and discuss a specific state or federal policy that pertains to case management with your selected field/population.

Part II: Needs and services analysis

Identify and discuss the common biopsychosocial needs that are experienced by the clients in your selected field/population.

Identify specific common services/providers/programs that are used in the state of Maryland to meet the needs of the clients.

Part III: Field/site visit and interview with a practicing case manager

Choose an actual case management program in your chosen area and a practicing case manager in that program. You will gather information about what the case manager actually does (role).

Part IV: Skill/strategy design

Based on your interview, choose one of the nine generic case management functions to discuss in depth with respect to specific skills and change strategies for that client population.

Include, with Parts I-IV of your portfolio, a specific list of references and resources you used in completing the assignment.

PORTFOLIO GUIDELINES

Part I: Policy Background (understanding the service delivery system)

Case management is typically only one part of a larger array of services and programs that form the so-called human services system in a particular field (child welfare, health, aging, disabilities, etc.), or for particular vulnerable groups (domestic violence victims, persons with AIDS, prisoners, etc.). Most services and programs receive public money for at least some of what they do. Thus they must respond to the decisions and decision-making process that is public policy.

To work in case management the professional must have a working knowledge of the public policies that shape and fund services and programs, and that determine their overall goals. This knowledge is essential to understand the expectations, supports, and pressures on the case management program and the individual case manager. It also is essential for making skillful use of the available service environment on behalf of each client.

For this part of your case management analysis, you are to research, read, and discuss a specific policy that pertains to the field/target population that will be the focus of your portfolio. Adhere to the following guidelines to complete Part I.

1. Do background reading/interviewing to determine a current public policy that is shaping/funding services, including case management, in your chosen area.

2. Read relevant parts of the policy (court decision, law, regulation) or a professional article discussing and interpreting the policy. Think about the implications of the policy for case management practice.

3. Prepare a written summary of no more than 3 pages.

   a. Identify the policy. Explain the overall policy in your own words.

   b. Explain what the policy says, if anything, about case management.

   c. Discuss your ideas about the implications of the overall policy for case management programs and clients in this chosen area.

4. Prepare a bibliography/reference page, citing the resources (in APA format) that you used for this section.

Part II: Needs and Services (understanding your clients and resources)

In this section you are increasing your knowledge of the special needs, characteristics, and capacities of the target population of clients for your selected area, and of the resources that exist in the environment to help. Follow the guidelines below to prepare Part II of your portfolio.

1. Read a selection of recent (since 1992) professional journal articles that deal with your target population to identify key aspects of both their vulnerability and their strength.

2. Explore the resource environment in Maryland. What are the types of actual services that are out there to help? Do some digging.

3. Write up your findings in no more than 5 pages.

   a. Person. Summarize in your own words your conclusions about the general needs and capacities of your target group. Use a biopsychosocial framework to discuss both the nature of the vulnerability and strengths.

   b. Environment. Summarize the results of your investigation concerning environmental resources and opportunities. What gaps and/or barriers do there seem to be?

4. Prepare a bibliography/reference page citing the resources used for this section.

Part III: Field/Site Visit and Interview with a Case Manager (understanding the model of social work case management)

1. Identify the agency and program that you visit. Briefly describe how the case management program or case management service fits with the overall service mission of the agency.

2. Design a series of questions to ask the case manager that will allow you to get a clear picture of the role, functions, and tasks actually carried out. [It's not enough to simply ask the case manager, "What do you do?"] Use the questions as a guide to your interview. Don't be shy about asking, "Can you give me an example of that?"

3. Write up an account of your interview.

   a. Describe the case manager role in this agency and program as you understand it from your interview.

   b. Analyze the role in terms of Greene's "Key Features of Social Work Case Management Practice" (Vourlekis & Greene, p. 12). What are your conclusions about the similarities and differences of the role of the person you interviewed and this "ideal" model of social work case management practice? What factors explain the similarities and differences that you see?

4. Attach to your write-up the list of questions you developed before conducting the interview.

Part IV: Skill/Strategy Design (understanding the skilled work of case management)

1. Select one of the eight generic case management functions discussed in class.

2. Using the understanding gathered in your interview with a practicing case manager, describe and discuss in depth this one function as it is carried out in this real program.

3. Again, using the same one function, identify specific skills and strategies that are or would be important to successfully carrying out this function of case management. Please discuss and illustrate at least one specific skill and strategy for both the client level and the system level.

Please note: I do not expect you to ask the case manager you interview to do Part IV (smile!). Think about this. You are taking this class to learn concepts to guide practice and to identify them in real-life circumstances. When you have a good picture of the way the case manager operates, after your interview, I expect you to figure out which information relates to the different functions we are studying. Likewise, I want you to think about what it would be like to be practicing case management as your informant does, and to think about skills and strategies that would help.

Shippensburg University
Social Work Department
Shippensburg, PA

Course Title: Special Fields of Social Work: Health Settings (SWK 357)
Fall 1998

Course Instructor: Denise Anderson

DESCRIPTION

Extends and elaborates the generalist approach to social work practice to a special field of practice. The special field is studied through the examination of curricular areas: human behavior, practice, policy and services, research, and special populations. Special fields courses include but are not limited to: Domestic Violence Settings (SWK 350), Aging Settings (SWK 351), Child Welfare Settings (SWK 352), Mental Health Settings (SWK 354), Mental Retardation Settings (SWK 356), School Settings (SWK 358), and Substance Abuse Settings (SWK 359). Prerequisites: SWK 102, SWK 150, and SWK 250.

APPROACH

The purpose of this course is to introduce the students to the social worker's role in health care. The course will focus on three content areas: what social workers' role is in different health care settings (i.e., discharge planning in hospitals); historic and current policy that affect health care services; and current research in various health care–related issues (i.e., living wills, AIDS).

The course will include the use of lecture, class and small group discussion, field trips, guest speakers, research papers, exams, presentations, and other written assignments.

OBJECTIVES

Through this course of study students should be able to:
1. Understand past and present health care policies.
2. Understand the major roles and functions of social workers in health care settings.
3. Understand the different issues that social workers deal with in health care settings.
4. Demonstrate a thorough understanding of one selected issue in health care.

Competency Outcomes for this course:
1. Promote and advocate for access to empowerment and opportunity.
2. Demonstrate problem-solving approaches.
3. Apply the generalist approach on multi-levels of intervention in social work practice.

REQUIRED TEXT

Kerson, T., et al. (1997). *Social Work in Health Settings* (2nd ed.). Binghamton, NY: Haworth.

REQUIREMENTS

1. Exams - There will be a midterm and final exam. Each exam will include both objective and subjective questions. Total points=200 (100 for each exam)

2. Research paper - Students will form groups of three and will select a broad health care topic. Each student will then narrow the focus of that topic and independently write a 15-20 page, typed, double-spaced, APA-style research paper. Topics must be cleared by the professor prior to the start of the research. Total points=100

    Suggested topics

    Living wills

    Abuse of a specific population (i.e., elderly, child, etc.)

    AIDS

    Care of the elderly

    Teen pregnancy

    Drug or alcohol abuse

    Mental illness

3. Presentation - Students will be responsible for providing a group presentation of findings to the class to allow all students to learn about many topics. Presentations will be 30 minutes minimum and combine all three research findings. Total points=50

4. Reaction papers to field trip - Students are required to type a 2-3 page reaction of feelings and thoughts about their field trip to a health care facility. Total points=50

5. Book report - Students are required to read "Mama might be better off dead" (a required text) and write a 3-5 page book report. Total points=50

6. Attendance and participation - All students are expected to attend class each week and to participate in small and large group discussions. Total points=50

Grading System

    450–500= A

    400–449= B

    350–399= C

    300–349= D

    Below 300= F

All assignments must be submitted on the due date. Five points will be deducted for each day the assignment is late.

SCHEDULE

Week 1

Introduction and Overview of course

Evolution of current health care (Historic and current system)

Week 2
Hospital Social Work: Discharge Planning/Medical Surgical
Guest Speaker—John Reese, MA, Social Worker, Holy Spirit Hospital
Read: Text, Chapter 10

Week 3
Field Trip
Chambersburg Hospital—Susan Dooley
Menno Haven Nursing Home—Jaime Nye

Week 4
Panel of Speakers, "Changes in the Health Care Field: Managed Care/Ethics"
  John Reese

  Cynthia Howard, Director of SS, Community Mental Health

  Toni McMullen, Director of SS, Shippensburg Health Care Center

Week 5
Ethics in Health Care Settings
Guest Speaker—Susan Zeigler, Director of SS, Holy Spirit Hospital
Read: Text, Chapter 13

Week 6
Health Care for the Aging Population—Nursing Home/Home Health
Guest Speaker—Toni McMullen
Read: Text, Chapters 29–33

Week 7
Mental Health
Guest Speakers—Candace Highfield, LSW Community Mental Health
Amy Fabrizio, LSW - Teenline
Read: Text, Chapters 20–28
Assignment: Field Trip Reaction Papers due

Week 8
Midterm Exam

Week 9
Terminal Illness
Guest Speaker—Sherry Kennedy, BSW, Holy Spirit Hospital
Read: Text, Chapters 12 & 14

Week 10
HIV/AIDS and Health Care
Jenny Englerith, Director of HIV/AIDS Program—Keystone Health
Read: Text, Chapters 2 & 19
Assignment: Book Report Due

Week 11
Reproductive issues and social work
Guest Speaker—Leslie Wagner, BSW—Maternity Clinic
Read: Text, Chapter 1

Week 12
Rehabilitation Social Work
Guest Speaker—John Young, MSW, Social Worker
Assignment: Research Paper

Week 13
Group Presentations
Research Paper Due

Week 14
Group Presentations

Week 15
Final Exam (Comprehensive—including presentations)

ASSIGNMENT DETAILS

Book Report Guidelines

Each student is required to read 'Mama might be better off dead' (Abraham, 1994, University of Chicago Press) and write a 4-5 page report. This report will include:

- A brief summary of the book (approx. 2 pages)

- Your personal reaction (feelings) about the book content (approx. 2 pages)

- Your professional reaction (what would you do as a social worker) about the book content (approx. 1 page)

Research Paper Guidelines

Each group of three students must select a health care topic that is of current concern (ex., Pregnancy). Each student will then select a more specific topic (ex., Teen pregnancy, Infertility). The content of the 15-20 page, typed, double-spaced research paper should include:

    I. Introduction

    II. Description of problem

        A. Definition

        B. Prevalence

        C. Scope

        D. Target population

    III. Literature review

        A. History of problem

        B. Current solutions/practice methods pertaining to problem

    IV. Selection of method of practice

        A. Based upon current literature, what do you recommend as the most effective method of dealing with the problem?

    V. Conclusion

Guidelines for Healthcare Facility Visit

Each student will select a healthcare facility that he/she would like to visit (e.g.., nursing home, hospital, reproductive clinic, hospice).

You must schedule your visit with a social worker at the facility.

Each student will develop at least three questions (relevant to the practice setting, e.g., 'What are your primary roles at this facility?') for the social worker.

Following the visit, you must write a 2-3 page reaction paper which will include: a general description of the agency, the answers to the questions asked, and your personal feelings about working in that setting/agency of social work.

Group Presentation Guidelines

Each team of three students will present research findings at a conference (classroom) related to the topic (ex., Conference on Pregnancy: Solutions for Social Work Practice).

The students will integrate the findings from all three topics and report to the other students in a 30-minute minimum presentation.

Presentation will be graded on relevance and clarity of content, creativity of presentation, and the ability to integrate each student's material.

BIBLIOGRAPHY

Bendor, S. (1987). The clinical challenge of hospital-based social work practice. *Social Work in Health Care, 13*(2), 25-33.

Cox, C. (1992). Expanding social worker's role in home care: An ecological perspective. *Social Work, 37*(2), 179-183.

Ellman, I. (1990, Jan/Feb.). Can others exercise an incapacitated patient's right to die? *Hastings Center Report,* 47-50.

Greenfield, D., Diamond, M., Breslin, R., & DeCherney, A. (1986). Infertility and the new reproductive technique: A role for social work. *Social Work in Health Care, 12*(2), 71-81.

Googin, B., & Davidson, B. (1993). The organization as client: Broadening the concept of employee assistance programs. *Social Work, 38*(4), 380-387.

Indyk, D., Belville, R., LaChapelle, S., Gorden, G., & Dewart, T. (1993). A community-based approach to HIV case management. *Social Work, 38*(4), 477-484.

Lotz, N., & DuChainey, D. (1988). Reestablishing a coordinated care program: Home health services. *Social Work in Health Settings,* 373-387.

Nacman, M. (1977). Social work in health settings: A historical review. *Social Work in Health Care, 2*(4), 7-21.

Reamer, F. G. (1990). *Ethical dilemmas in social service* (2nd ed.). New York: Columbia University Press.

Reamer, F. G. (1993). AIDS and social work: The ethics and civil liberties agenda. *Social Work, 38*(4), 412-419.

Starr, P. (1982). *The social transforming medicine.* New York: Basic Books.

Stevens, R. (1989). *In sickness and in wealth: American hospitals in the 20th century.* New York: Basic Books.

Wells, P. (1993). Preparing for sudden death: Social work in the emergency room. *Social Work, 38*(4), 339-342.

Wolf, S. (1990, Jan./Feb.). Nancy Beth Cruzan: In no voice at all. *Hastings Center Report,* 8-46.

Roberts Wesleyan College
Master of Social Work Program
Rochester, NY

Course Title: Social Work Issues in Health Care (SWK 663)
                                Fall 1998

Course Instructor: David A. Sherwood

OVERVIEW

The MSW curriculum at Roberts is organized around three frameworks. The first framework is a conceptual framework which provides coherence to the program objectives. This framework consists of 10 key areas: professional development, values and ethics, diversity, social and economic justice, at-risk populations, human behavior and the social environment, social welfare policy and services, social work practice, research, and field experience. Each course and each assignment in some way addresses content in one of these 10 areas.

The second framework is an overall philosophical framework referred to as the Spiritually Enriched Ecological Systems perspective. An ecological systems perspective essentially holds that life is best understood as a symbiotic relationship between persons and their environments. To this widely used framework, the Roberts program adds the spiritual perspective, i.e., human existence involves a search for meaning.

The third framework, a unifying practice model, is referred to as the Strengths Oriented Life Model. This practice model combines the Life Model and the Strengths Perspective. The Life Model highlights life transitions, environmental stressors, and maladaptive interpersonal processes, while the Strengths Perspective emphasizes the concept of empowerment. At the foundation level, students are taught generalist practice preparing them to work with systems of various sizes using the Strengths Oriented Life Model. Advanced practice skills build on the Strengths Oriented Life Model using a Family-Centered Practice Model or Interlocking Theories Framework in the Child and Family or Physical and Mental Health concentration, respectively, as the unifying practice frameworks.

CONTRIBUTION OF THIS COURSE

This course gives major attention to the following Concentration Program Objectives: HBSE, Social Work and Social Welfare, Policy Analysis, and Intervention. In addition, the course addresses the following in a significant way: Critical Thinking, Communication, Values and Ethics, Diversity, At-Risk Populations, Low-Income, Justice, and Research Consumer, HBSE, Policy Analysis, and Social Action.

Following is the complete wording of the Concentration Program Objectives that this course addresses. The notations of Major, Significant, and Important give some indication of how much weight that particular objective has in this course. Major indicates a primary thrust of the course. Significant indicates a prominent but less than major attention. The Important category indicates this objective is addressed but is not the focus of direct evaluation. The number indicates the specific Program Objective.

Demonstrate a critical understanding of theories relevant to assessment of children and families or persons needing physical/mental health services consistent with a Spiritually Enriched Ecological Systems perspective. **(#11. HBSE, Major)**

Demonstrate an awareness of the history of child and family or physical/mental health services, the state of present services, the direction in which services are changing, and the role of social work in providing services. **(# 12. Social Work & Welfare, Major)**

Demonstrate an ability to analyze historical and current child and family social policy. **(# 13. Policy Analysis, Major)**

Demonstrate an ability to identify theories and strategies and to provide appropriate advanced practice intervention to children and families using the Family-Centered Practice Model as the unifying framework or to persons needing physical/mental health services utilizing Interlocking Theories Practice as the unifying practice framework. **(#16. Intervention, Major)**

Demonstrate the ability to apply critical thinking skills to advanced practice social work knowledge, values, and skills relating to children and families or persons needing physical/mental health services. **(#1. Critical Thinking, Major)**

Demonstrate advanced written and verbal communication skills. **(#3, Communication, Major)**

Demonstrate the ability to critically analyze value and ethical issues and resolve dilemmas relative to advanced practice with children and families or to persons needing physical/mental health services. **(#5. Values & Ethics, Significant)**

Demonstrate the ability to incorporate diversity knowledge and sensitivity in assessment and intervention with children and families or persons needing physical/mental health services. **(#6. Diversity, Significant)**

Demonstrate the ability to incorporate knowledge about the dynamics and consequences of discrimination, oppression, social and economic injustice, as well as empowerment, reconciliation, and justice in assessment and intervention with practice situations involving children and families or persons needing physical/mental health services. **(#8. Justice, Significant)**

Demonstrate the ability to incorporate knowledge about at-risk populations in assessment and intervention with practice situations involving children and families or persons needing physical/mental health services including factors related to race and ethnicity, gender, and sexual orientation. **(#9. At-Risk Populations, Significant)**

Demonstrate an ability to incorporate knowledge about low-income populations when providing services to children and families or persons needing physical/mental health services. **(#10. Low-Income, Significant)**

Demonstrate an ability to incorporate literature relevant to practice with children and families or persons needing physical/mental services including empirical research. **(#17. Research Consumer, Significant)**

Demonstrate the professional use of self when working with children and families or with persons needing physical/mental health services. **(#2. Use of Self, Important)**

Demonstrate the ability to use the empowering aspects of spirituality and religion and reduce dysfunctional aspects when engaged in advanced practice with children and families or persons needing physical/mental health services. (**#7. Spirituality & Religion, Important**)

Demonstrate an ability to develop action strategies that would bring positive changes related to children and families utilizing empowerment to bring about reconciliation and social justice. (**#14. Social Action, Important**)

Demonstrate an ability to develop action strategies that would bring positive changes related to children and families or persons needing physical/mental health services using the Spiritually Enriched Ecological Systems perspective as the unifying practice framework. (**#15. Assessment, Important**)

COURSE DESCRIPTION

The course explores the ecology of social work in health care at the threshold of the 21st century. This is accomplished by examining an array of practice contexts and issues which affect the practice of social work in health care. Of particular concern is the dynamism which managed care has given social work within the health care enterprise. Students will analyze the resultant diffusion of boundaries between mental and physical health care, and explore the challenges involved in moving toward a more seamless reformulation of social work methods and processes within health care.

COURSE OBJECTIVES

Cognitive

1. Understand how managed care is reshaping the role of social work in health care at the threshold of the 21st century.
2. Explore the seamless, more generic nature of physical and mental health social work in the era of managed care.
3. Understand how the array of physical health care challenges (e.g., specific types of physical illnesses, practice contexts, organizational structures, political/economic dynamics) serve as contexts for health care social work purposes and functions.
4. Understand how the array of physical health care challenges (i.e., specific types of physical illnesses, practice contexts, organizational structures, political/economic dynamics) guide the selection, and use of particular theories by exploring issues of the limits of utility, boundaries, and functionality.
5. Understand the intra-systemic and inter-systemic social and organizational issues which impact social work roles in health care.
6. Understand the etiological issues and practice implications related to a range of health care challenges.

Affective

1. Appreciate the creative energy which managed care can supply to social work in health care at the threshold of the 21st century.
2. Appreciate the importance of the context of various physical health care challenges as critical to giving shape and definition to social work roles in health care settings.
3. Appreciate the importance of social work expertise in negotiating internal and external systems on behalf of clients as critical to healing and health.
4. Value the necessity of making health care systems more humane and caring for all clients, and accessible for clients who are economically compromised.

5. Gain confidence in ability to manage and adapt to change and be able to value the importance of social work leadership within health care settings.

Behavioral

1. Be able to reframe social work roles in health care in the context of systemic analysis and problem-solving to become "systems expediters."
2. Begin formulation of a repertoire of leadership strategies appropriate for social work in health care in the era of managed care.
3. Use learning from course to inform use of self as vital part of interdisciplinary health care teams.
4. Utilize social work values, knowledge, and skills to assess practice issues in health care and to develop effective intervention strategies.
5. Be able to understand and use medical terminology.

TEXTS

Required

Abraham, L. K. (1993). *Mama might be better off dead: The failure of health care in urban America.* Chicago: University of Chicago Press.

Dhooper, S. S. (1997). *Social work in health care in the 21st century.* Thousand Oaks, CA: Sage.

Thomas, C. L. (Ed.). (1997). *Tabor's cyclopedic medical dictionary, 18th ed.* Philadelphia: F. A. Davis Company.

Recommended

Corcoran, K., & Vandiver, V. (1996). *Maneuvering the maze of managed care.* New York: Free Press.

Davidson, K. W., & Clarke, S. (1990). *Social work in health care: A handbook for practice* (Volumes I & II). New York: Haworth.

Jackson, V. H. (Ed.). (1995). *Managed care resource guide for social workers in agency settings.* Washington, DC: NASW Press.

CLASSROOM COMPORTMENT AND ACADEMIC EXPECTATIONS

General Comments: Classroom activities will include lecture, discussion, and occasional guests, but will primarily emphasize a student-led seminar format in which you will present the results of your research and thinking to your colleagues and lead them in discussion. When you are not presenting, you are expected to 1) read and think about each reading assignment prior to class; 2) reflect on the usefulness of the material; and 3) participate freely and constructively in class. While occasional lateness or absence is inevitable, a pattern of either may affect your grade. Likewise, while silence is appropriate at times, excessive non-participation may affect the final grade.

Writing Policy: Academic writing requires a strong culture of careful documentation of the use of sources, both to ensure intellectual integrity and to provide the apparatus for scholarly work by others using your materials. You should employ thorough academic documentation of sources of information, ideas, and direct quotes. The program requires you write using APA documentation style.

Plagiarism, inadequate documentation of sources, and excessive dependence on the language of your sources (even when you document them) are completely unacceptable. It is not appropriate to submit the same or similar work for more than one course or assignment unless it has been documented, discussed with me, and approved. (However, it is quite appropriate to design a series of projects for more than one course around issues that relate to your own learning objectives.)

The best way to do research is the old-fashioned way—take notes using note cards (or the equivalent), carefully getting accurate bibliographic information, jotting down key ideas and information (and the pages you found them on), and collecting a few strategic direct quotes when the author makes the point you want in a particularly striking or effective way. Then when you sit down to write (using pencil or computer), you can organize your material in a variety of ways to serve your purposes, have the information you need at hand, and be able to liven up your paper with good quotations. There is no shortcut to good scholarship. The research will serve your goals and thought process, and, as a significant bonus, you won't be tempted to cheat. A recipe for poor writing, poor scholarship, and the development of poor character is to lay a bunch of articles and books in front of you on the table and proceed to try to paste some semblance of a paper together.

For additional information about writing and critical thinking, see the Student Handbook.

Honesty: Trust and integrity are essential to all good relationships, including educational and professional ones. This is particularly fundamental in a Christian context. Although dishonesty is ultimately simply self-defeating, since the College is in the position of certifying work through granting grades, academic credit, and finally professional degrees, the highest standards of integrity must be maintained. I assume that all work is entirely yours and that any variation from this or assistance received (quite appropriate in many cases) must be clearly documented and explained. Since I assume honesty, it is relatively easy for the student who chooses to be dishonest to take advantage of this. However, I am a skilled reader and should this principle of intellectual responsibility be violated, the normal result is an NC for the course based on the serious breach of ethics involved.

Grading Policy: My general policy is to require a substantial amount of work but to assure you of a reasonably good grade if you do it. Solid work will receive a grade in the B range. On the other hand, it is relatively difficult to achieve an A. An A represents the kind of consistently outstanding achievement that is uncommon, or it becomes meaningless.

An "A" indicates the paper excelled in both the level of thinking and in the writing. A "B" indicates acceptable thinking and writing but suggests one or both aspects could be improved. A grade lower than "B" indicated either one or both of the areas is not up to graduate level performance. Papers which do not indicate graduate level work (below a B-) may be redone one time.

Due Dates: Assignments such as papers are due on the specified date. Requests for extensions must be based on significant extenuating circumstances and must be discussed with me before the assignment is due. My normal policy is to deduct one percentage point from the assigned grade per day late (e.g., a grade of 96% becomes 95%, then 94%, etc.). Sometimes a couple of points is a reasonable price to pay for a couple of needed extra days. But they begin to add up.

Incompletes: An incomplete grade for the course is normally given only after you have established with me, before the end of the term, that your work is incomplete for good cause and a plan has been agreed upon for the completion of the work. It is your responsibility to make up any incomplete work within the agreed time. Incompletes are very rare and should never be taken for granted.

Book Return Policy: Please be aware of the book return policy when buying books at the bookstore. Returned books are only accepted for two reasons: the student has changed courses or the course is cancelled; and, the student bought books for the wrong course.

ASSIGNMENTS

Managed Care Paper (20%):

Write a 6–10 page paper exploring the issue of managed care and its impact on health care generally and social work services particularly, using your field placement setting as the primary case in point. What does "managed care" mean to your agency now? What is it likely to mean in the future?

Explore the impact of managed care at three levels:

1. How it will reconfigure service delivery.
2. How it is changing the professional culture of the agency.
3. What tensions and concerns it raises.

Analyze possible positive benefits as well as negative outcomes of managed care in both health and mental health care, examining similarities and differences between health and mental health. Your paper should make use of recent and current literature as well as agency materials and interviews with informed persons.

Program objectives on which this assignment will be evaluated include: Critical Thinking, Communication, Values & Ethics, Justice, At-Risk Populations, Low-Income, Social Work & Welfare, Policy Analysis, Intervention, and Research Consumer.

Health Care Social Work Practice Context (Paper = 25%; Presentation = 10%):

Write an 8–12 page paper and do a seminar presentation in which you explore and analyze a particular social work practice context in a major type of health care setting (acute care, ambulatory care, illness prevention/health promotion, long-term/community care).

Analyze how the social work purpose and function is uniquely configured by the particular systemic context. Clearly identify practice issues related to the client population served, interdisciplinary interactions, inter- and intra-systemic dynamics, and how these issues inform or challenge social work practice. Strategize regarding how social workers might exercise leadership in optimizing the social work role and services to meet the goal of enhancing the well-being of clients and assuring a socially just service delivery system. Analyze the current and emerging reality and strategize how it might be made better.

You will be responsible to present your chosen context to the rest of the class and lead a discussion of it. You will have about 45 minutes total for presentation and discussion and you may organize this in any way you believe would be most effective, including handouts, visuals, prepared questions, role-play, multimedia spectacles, fireworks, or feasts (no orgies, please). At minimum prepare a 1–2 page handout of key information and bibliographical resources for your colleagues.

In the interests of diversity and breadth of contexts presented, normally no more than one presentation can be on the same specific context (e.g., renal dialysis patients in ambulatory care), but you may team up with another presenter in the same general context (e.g., ambulatory care). In such cases, plan your presentations in such a way as to highlight commonalities and differences. We will follow the principle of first-come-first-served to achieve justice in regard to topics. The sooner you identify your preferred context to explore and notify me about it, the more likely you are to get your first choice.

Program objectives on which this assignment will be evaluated include: Critical Thinking, Communication, Diversity, Justice, At-Risk Populations, Low-Income, HBSE, Social Work & Welfare, Policy Analysis, Intervention, and Research Consumer.

Social Work in Health Care Issue (Paper = 25%; Presentation = 10%):

Write a 8–12 page paper and do a seminar presentation on an issue or intervention in health care social work practice of particular interest to you, critically exploring it in depth, using both formal and informal resources. Relate your discussion to the Interlocking Theories Practice Model and the Spiritually Enriched Ecological Systems perspective. Reflect on your own goals and how the materials from this course and other courses in the health and mental health concentration are informing your development.

Introduce the basic nature of your issue. It is usually best to choose an issue which has an "edge" to it—some sort of controversy, competing viewpoints, legitimate (and not-so-legitimate) values in tension with each other. Do a careful, critical review of the literature, summarizing key findings and pointing out both significant areas of understanding and progress and areas where study has been lacking or inadequately done. Interview knowledgeable persons and seek unpublished resources and incorporate this material into your discussion. Combine your research with your own critical thinking to discuss the implications of your issue for social work practice, particularly emphasizing the implications for intervention.

You will be responsible to present your chosen issue to the rest of the class and lead a discussion of it. You will have about 45 minutes total for presentation and discussion and you may organize this in any way you believe would be most effective, including handouts, visuals, prepared questions, role-play, multimedia spectacles, fireworks, or feasts (no orgies, please). At minimum prepare a 1–2 page handout of key information and bibliographical resources for your colleagues.

In the interests of diversity and breadth of contexts presented, normally no more than one presentation can be on the same specific issue or intervention, but you may team up with another with a related issue. In such cases, plan your presentations in such a way as to highlight commonalities and differences. We will follow the principle of first-come-first-served to achieve justice in regard to topics. The sooner you identify your preferred issue to explore and notify me about it, the more likely you are to get your first choice.

Program objectives on which this assignment will be evaluated include: Critical Thinking, Communication, Values & Ethics, Diversity, At-Risk Populations, Low-Income, HBSE, Social Work & Welfare, Policy Analysis, Intervention, and Research Consumer.

GRADING SUMMARY

There will be no exams in this class. The grades will be assigned based on the following:

Managed Care Paper	20%
Health Care Social Work Practice Context Paper and Presentation	35%
(Paper = 25%; Presentation = 10%)	
Social Work in Health Care Issue Paper and Presentation	35%
(Paper = 25%; Presentation = 10%)	
Preparation, Participation, Attendance	10%

A: 96-100%, A-: 92-95%, B+: 87-91%, B: 83-86%, B-: 80-82%, C+: 77-79%, C: 73-76%, C-: 70-72%, D+: 67-69%, D: 60-66%, F: below 60%. Note that any course receiving a grade below B- must be retaken.

In addition to receiving a grade for each assignment and for the course as indicated above, an Objective Subscale Outcome Measure score from 0–10 will be assigned for each program objective identified in the assignment. (See the Student Handbook for a list of the objectives and an explication of the terms.) The scores for each program objective will be combined with the scores from the same objectives in other assignments in this course and in other courses. Continuation in the program requires maintaining satisfactory averages in all of the program objectives as outlined in the Student Handbook.

1	2	3	4	5	6	7	8	9	10
D	C-	C	C+	B-	B	B+	A-	A	A+

CALENDAR AND ASSIGNMENTS
(see Bibliography for complete reference on readings)

Session 1

Overview.

Class orientation.

Traditional foundations.

Begin sign-up for contexts, issues.

Session 2

Changing environment of social work in health care.

Abraham (1993), 1-259; Dhooper (1997), 1-48.

Session 3

Managed care.

Corcoran & Vandiver (1996), 1-42; Jackson (1995), 2.1–2.15, 3.1–3.5, 4.1–4.10, 5.1–5.7; Perloff (1996), 189-195.

Session 4

Managed care.

Managed care paper due.

Berger, et al. (1996), 167-177; Browne, et al. (1996), 267-276; Keigher (1997), 149-155; Strom-Gottfried & Corcoran (1998), 109-119.

Session 5

Contexts: Acute care.

Begin contexts presentations/discussions.

Dhooper (1997), 49-55, 95-101, 131-170; Berger (1990), 77-93; Berkman, Bonander, et al. (1996), 115-135; Sands, et al. (1990), 55-72.

Session 6

Contexts: Ambulatory care.

Context presentations/discussions.

Dhooper (1997), 56-70, 102-107, 171-205; Berkman, Shearer, et al. (1996), 1-20; DeChillo (1993), 104-115; Shera (1996), 196-201.

Session 7

Contexts: Illness prevention/health promotion.

Context presentations/discussions.

Dhooper (1997), 71-83, 108-114, 206-248; Hayes & Gantt (1992), 53-67; Bender & Hart (1986), 52-58.

Session 8

Contexts: Long-term care/community care.

Context presentations/discussions.

Dhooper (1997), 84-94, 115-119, 249-291; Vourlekis, et al. (1995), 81-93; Simmons (1994), 35-46; Pray (1992), 71-79; Vourlekis, et al. (1992), 45-70.

Session 9

Issues exploration.
Case management.

Begin issue presentations/discussions.

Netting (1992), 160-164; Morrow-Howell (1992), 119-131; Netting & Williams (1996), 216-224.

Session 10

Issues exploration.
Discharge planning.

Issues presentations/discussions.

Oktay, et al. (1992), 290-298; Blumenfield & Rosenberg (1988), 31-48.

Session 11

Issues exploration.
Organization, management of health care social services.

Issues presentations/discussions.

Bixby (1995), 1-20; Globerman, et al. (1996), 178-188; Mayer (1995), 61-72.

Session 12

Issues exploration.
Ethics.

Issues presentations/discussion.

Davidson & Davidson (1996), 208-215; Wesley (1996), 115-121; Cummings & Cockerham (1997), 101-108; Foster, et al. (1993), 15-38.

Session 13

Issues exploration.
Diversity.

Issues presentations/discussion.

Congress & Lyons (1992), 81-96; Clifford (1994), 35-59; York (1987), 31-45; Aguilar (1997), 83-84.

BIBLIOGRAPHY

Abraham, L. K. (1994). *Mama might be better off dead: The failure of health care in urban America.* Chicago: University of Chicago Press.

Abramson, J. S. (1990). Enhancing patient participation: Clinical strategies in the discharge planning process. *Social Work in Health Care, 14*(4), 53-71.

Abramson, J. S., & Mizrahi, T. 1996). When social workers and physicians collaborate: Positive and negative interdisciplinary experiences. *Social Work, 41*(3), 270-280.

Abramson, M. (1983). A model for organizing an ethical analysis of the discharge planning process. *Social Work in Health Care, 9*(1), 45-52.

Abramson, M. (1990). Ethics and technological advances: Contributions of social work practice. *Social Work in Health Care, 15*(2), 77-93.

Abramson, M. (1996). Toward a more holistic understanding of ethics in social work. *Social Work in Health Care, 23*(2), 1-14.

Aday, L. (1993). *At risk in America: The health and health care needs of vulnerable populations in the United States.* San Francisco: Jossey-Bass.

Aguilar, M. A. (1997). Re-engineering social work's approach to holistic healing. *Health and Social Work, 22*(2), 83-84.

Allison, H., Gripton, J., & Rodway, M. (1983). Social work services as a component of palliative care with terminal cancer patients. *Social Work in Health Care, 8*(4), 29-44.

Aronson, J. (1966). *Inside managed care: Family therapy in a changing environment.* New York: Brunner/Mazel.

Atkatz, J. (1994). Discharge planning for homeless patients: A social work practice dilemma. Doctoral dissertation, Yeshiva University.

Barth, R. P., et al. (1994). *From child abuse to permanency planning: Child welfare services pathways and placements.* New York: Aldine de Gruyter.

Beaver, M. (1992). *Clinical social work practice with the elderly: Primary, secondary, and tertiary intervention.* Belmont, CA: Wadsworth.

Beckerman, N. (1991). Ethical dilemmas facing hospital social workers and policy and practice implications. Doctoral dissertation, Yeshiva University.

Beckman, D., & Bailey, D. (1966). *Strategies for working with families of young children with disabilities.* Baltimore, MD: Paul H. Brookes.

Bender, C., & Hart, J. (1986). Rural health promotion: Bailiwick for social work. *Health and Social Work, 11*(1), 52-58.

Bendor, B. J. (1987). The clinical challenge of hospital based social work practice. *Social Work in Health Care, 13*(2), 25-34.

Berger, C. S. (1990). Enhancing social work influence in the hospital: Identifying sources of power. *Social Work in Health Care, 15*(2), 77-93.

Berger, C. S., Cayner, J., Jensen, G., Mizrahi, T., Scesny, A., & Trachtenberg, J. (1996). The changing scene of social work in hospitals: A report of a national study by the society for social work administrators in health care and NASW. *Health and Social Work, 21*(4), 167-177.

Bergman, A. S., Contro, N., & Zivetz, N. (1984). Clinical social work in a medical setting. *Social Work in Health Care, 9*(3), 1-12.

Berkman, B. (1996). The emerging health care world: Implications for social work practice and education. *Social Work, 41*(5), 541-551.

Berkman, B., Bonander, E., Kemler, B., Rubinger, M., Rutchick, I., & Silverman, P. (1996). Social work in the academic medical center: Advanced training—a necessity. *Social Work in Health Care, 24*(1/2), 115-135.

Berkman, B., Campion, E., Swagerty, E., & Goldman, M. (1983). Geriatric consultation team: Alternate approach to social work discharge planning. *Journal of Gerontological Social Work, 5*(3), 77-88.

Berkman, B., Shearer, S., Simmons, W., White, M., Robinson, M., Sampson, S., Holmes, W., Allison, D., & Thompson, J. (1996). Ambulatory elderly patients or primary care physicians: Functional, psychosocial and environmental predictors of need for social work case management. *Social Work in Health Care, 22*(3), 1-20.

Berry, M. (1994). *Keeping families together.* New York: Garland.

Biegel, D. E., Shore, B. K., & Gordon, E. (1984). *Building support networks for the elderly: Theory and applications.* Beverly Hills, CA: Sage.

Bixby, N. B. (1995). Crisis or opportunity: A healthcare social work director's response to change. *Social Work in Health Care, 20*(4), 1-20.

Black, R. B. (1989). Challenges for social work as a core profession in cancer services. *Social Work in Health Care, 14*(1), 1-13.

Borenstein, D. B. (1996). Does managed care permit appropriate use of psychotherapy? *Psychiatric Services, 47,* 971-974.

Blumenfield, S. (1992). Teaching geriatric social work in health care—The what, why, or how of a complex process. *Journal of Gerontological Social Work, 18*(3/4), 55-71.

Blumenfield, S., & Rosenberg, G. (1988). Towards a network of social health services: Redefining discharge planning and expanding the social work domain. *Social Work in Health Care, 13*(4), 31-48.

Bodenheimer, T. S. (1996). *Managed care, capitation, and health care organization in today's health care environment.* Boston: Allyn and Bacon.

Bodenheimer, T. S., & Brumbach, K. (1998). *Understanding health policy: A clinical approach* (2nd ed.). Stamford, CT: Appleton and Lange.

Borland, J., & Jones, A. (1980). Referral patterns for social work services ambulatory care setting. *Journal of Applied Social Sciences, 5*(1), 19-33.

Boyd-Franklin, N., Steiner, G. L., & Boland, M. (1995). *Children, families, and HIV/AIDS: Psychosocial and therapeutic issues.* New York: Guilford.

Bradey, R. (1985). Crisis social work intervention with families experiencing sudden infant death. *Australian Social Work, 38*(2), 35-37.

Brantlinger, E. (1995). *Sterilization of people with mental disabilities: Issues, perspectives, and cases.* Westport, CT: Auburn House.

Brennan, J., & Kaplan, C. (1993, March). Setting new standards for social work case management. *Hospital and Community Psychiatry,* 219-222.

Brey, H., & Jarvis, J. (1983). Life change: Adjusting to continuous ambulatory peritoneal dialysis. *Health and Social Work, 8*(3), 203-209.

Brikner, P. W., et al. (1987). *Long-term health care: Providing a spectrum of services to the aged.* New York: Basic Books.

Bross, D., & et al. (1988). *The new child protection team handbook.* New York: Garland.

Browne, C. V., Smith, M., Ewalt, P. L., & Walker, D. D. (1996). Advancing social work practice in health care settings: A collaborative partnership for continuing education. *Health and Social Work, 21*(4), 267-276.

Bull, N., (Ed.). (1993). *Aging in rural America.* Newbury Park, CA: Sage.

Bushnell, G. M. (1993). *Final choices: To live or to die in an age of medical technology.* New York: Insight.

Callahan, J. (1996). Documentation of client dangerousness in a managed care environment. *Health and Social Work, 21*(4), 202-207.

Caplan, A. L. (1992). *If I were a rich man could I buy a pancreas? And other essays on the ethics of health care.* Bloomington, IN: Indiana University Press.

Carlton, T. O. (1984). *Clinical social work in health care settings.* New York: Springer.

Carstensen, L., Edelstein, B., & Dornbrand, L. (1966). *The practical handbook of clinical gerontology.* Thousand Oaks, CA: Sage.

Cash, T., & Valentine, D. (1987). A decade of adult protective services: Case characteristics. *Journal of Gerontological Social Work, 10*(3/4), 47-60.

Challis, D., & Hugman, R. (1993, August). Editorial: Community care, social work and social care. *British Journal of Social Work,* 319-328.

Christ, G. H. (1996). School and agency collaboration in a cost-conscious health care environment. *Social Work in Health Care, 24*(1/2), 53-72.

Clifford, M. W. (1994). Social work treatment with children, adolescents, and families exposed to religious and Satanic cults. *Social Work in Health Care, 20*(2), 35-59.

Cohen, J., & Wannamaker, M. (1966). *Expressive arts for the very disabled and handicapped for all ages* (2nd ed.). Springfield, IL: Charles C. Thomas.

Combs-Orme, T. (1990). *Social work practice in maternal and child health.* New York: Springer.

Congress, E. P., & Lyons, B. P. (1992). Cultural differences in health beliefs: Implications for social work practice in health care settings. *Social Work in Health Care, 17*(3), 81-96.

Coper, P. (1995). The next shift: Managed care. *Public Health Reports, 110,* 682-683.

Cook, C. A. L., Chadiha, L., Schmidt, B., Holloway, J., & Satterwhite, J. L. (1992). High social risk screening mechanisms: Patient characteristics as predictors of social work utilization in the VA. *Social Work in Health Care, 16*(4), 101-117.

Corcoran, K., & Vandiver, V. (1996). *Maneuvering the maze of managed care.* New York: Free Press.

Cornelius, D. S. (1994). Managed care and social work: Constructing a context and a response. *Social Work in Health Care, 20*(1), 47-63.

Cummings, S. M., & Cockerham, C. (1997). Ethical dilemmas in discharge planning for patients with Alzheimer's disease. *Health and Social Work, 22*(2), 101-108.

Daniels, K. R. (1989). Psychosocial factors for couples awaiting in vitro fertilization. *Social Work in Health Care, 14*(2), 81-98.

Daniels, N., & Sabin, J. (1998). Last chance therapies and managed care: Pluralism, fair procedures, and legitimacy. *Hastings Center Report, 28*(2), 27-41.

Davidson, K. W., & Clarke, S. (1990). *Social work in health care: A handbook for practice* (Vols. I & II). Binghamton, NY: Haworth.

Davidson, J. R., & Davidson, T. (1996). Confidentiality and managed care: Ethical and legal concerns. *Health and Social Work, 21*(4), 208-215.

Davis, A. G. (1982). *Children in clinics: A sociological analysis of medical social work with children.* New York: Tavistock.

Davis, K. E. (1996). Primary health care and severe mental illness: The need for national and state policy. *Health and Social Work, 21*(2), 83-87.

DeChillo, N. (1993, February). Collaboration between social workers and families of patients with mental illness. *Families in Society: The Journal of Contemporary Human Services,* 104-115.

Dhooper, S. S. (1997). *Social work in health care in the 21st century.* Thousand Oaks, CA: Sage.

Dobrof, J. (1991). DRGs and the social worker's role in discharge planning. *Social Work in Health Care, 16*(2), 37-54.

Dobrof, R. (Ed.). (1987). *Ethnicity and gerontological social work.* Binghamton, NY: Haworth.

Dobrof, R., & Litwak, E. (1977). *Maintenance of family ties of long-term care patients: Theory and guide to practice.* Rockville, MD: Public Health Service, Alcohol, Drug Abuse, and Mental Health Administration.

Dworkin, J. (1997). Social workers and national health care: Are there lessons from Great Britain? *Health and Social Work, 22*(2), 117-123.

Egan, M., & Kadushin, G. (1995). Competitive allies: Rural nurses' and social workers' perceptions of the social work role in the hospital setting. *Social Work in Health Care, 20*(3), 1-23.

Ell, K. (1996, Nov.). Social work and health care practice and policy: A psychosocial research agenda. *Social Work,* 583-592.

Ell, K., & Northen, H. (1990). *Families and health care: Psychosocial practice.* New York: Aldine de Gruyter.

Erwin, K. (1966). *Group techniques for aging adults: Putting geriatric skills enhancement into practice.* Bristol, PA: Taylor and Francis.

Estes, C. L., Swan, J. H., et al. *The long-term care crisis: Elders trapped in the no care zone.* Newbury Park, CA: Sage.

Estes, R. J. (Ed.). (1984). *Health care and the social services: Social work practice in health care.* St. Louis: W. H. Green.

Fahs, M., & Wade, K. (1996). An economic analysis of two models of hospital care for AIDS patients: Implications for hospital discharge planning. *Social Work in Health Care, 22*(4), 21-34.

Faller, K. C. (1987). *Child sexual abuse: An interdisciplinary manual for diagnosis, case management, and treatment.* New York: Columbia University Press.

Feldman, S., & Goldman, W., (Eds.). (1992). *Managed mental health services.* Springfield, IL: Charles C. Thomas.

Foster, L. W., Sharp, J. W., Scesny, A., McLellan, L., & Cotman, K. (1993). Bioethics: Social work's response and training needs. *Social Work in Health Care, 19*(1), 15-38.

Foster, Z., Hirsch, S., & Zaske, K. (1992). Social work role in developing and managing employee assistance programs in health care settings. *Social Work in Health Care, 16*(2), 81-95.

Fulmer, T. T., & O'Malley, T. A. (1987). *Inadequate care of the elderly: A health care perspective on abuse and neglect.* New York: Springer.

Furlong, R. M. (1986). The social worker's role on the institutional ethics committee. *Social Work in Health Care, 11*(4), 93-100.

Gallagher, S. K. (1994). *Older people giving care: Helping family and community.* Westport, CT: Auburn House.

Germain, C. B. (1984). *Social work practice in health care: An ecological perspective.* New York: Free Press.

Getzel, G. S. (1986). Social work groups in health care settings: Four emerging approaches. *Social Work in Health Care, 12*(1), 23-38.

Gillman, R., & Newman, B. (1996, March). Psychosocial concerns and strengths of women with HIV infection: An empirical study. *Families in Society,* 134-141.

Globerman, J., Davies, J., & MacKenzie-Walsh, S. (1996). Social work in restructuring hospitals: Meeting the challenge. *Health and Social Work, 21*(4), 178-188.

Goldman, W., & Feldman, S. (Eds.). (1993). *Managed mental health care.* San Francisco: Jossey-Bass.

Goldmeier, J. (1984). Ethical styles and ethical decisions in health settings. *Social Work in Health Care, 10*(1), 45-60.

Gray, S. (1966). *Health of native people of North America: A bibliography and guide to resources.* Metuchen, NJ: Scarecrow.

Greene, G. J., & Kruse, K. A. (1985). Social work in family practice: What are the prospects? *Social Work in Health Care, 11*(1), 45-62.

Greene, R., & Lewis, J. (1990, Summer). Curriculum for case management with the frail elderly: A Delphi study. *Arete,* pp. 32-45.

Greenfield, D., Diamond, M. P., Breslin, R. L., & DeCherney, A. (1986, Winter). Infertility and the new reproductive technology: A role for social work. *Social Work in Health Care,* 71-81.

Gross, R., Rabinowitz, J., Feldman, D., & Boerma, W. (1996). Primary health care physicians' treatment of psychosocial problems: Implications for social work. *Health and Social Work, 21*(2), 89-95.

Haber, D. (1984). Church based programs for black care givers of non-institutionalized elders. *Journal of Gerontological Social Work, 7*(4), 43-55.

Hall, S. R. (1996). The community-centered board model of managed care for people with developmental disabilities. *Health Care and Social Work, 21*(4), 225-229.

Hancock, B. L. (1990). *Social work with older people.* Englewood Cliffs, NJ: Prentice Hall.

Hayes, R., & Gantt, A. (1992). Patient psychoeducations: The therapeutic use of knowledge for the mentally ill. *Social Work in Health Care, 17*(1), 53-67.

Hoffman, M. A. (1966). *Counseling clients with HIV disease: Assessment, intervention, and prevention.* New York: Guilford.

Hunter, M. (1966). *Making peace with chronic pain: A whole life strategy.* New York: Brunner/Mazel.

Hymovich, D. P., & Hagopian, G. A. (1995). *Chronic illness in children and adults: A psychosocial approach.* Philadelphia: Saunders.

Jackson, V. H. (Ed.). (1995). *Managed care resource guide for social workers in agency settings.* Washington, DC: NASW Press.

James, C., & Studs, D. (1987, Summer). An ecological approach to defining discharge planning in social work. *Social Work in Health Care, 12*(4), 47-59.

Jones, K. (1988). *Experience in mental health: Community care and social policy.* Newbury Park, CA: Sage.

Julia, M. C. (Ed.). (1995). *Multicultural awareness in the health care professions.* Boston: Allyn and Bacon.

Kaplan, L. (1997). *Consumer's guide to New York's managed care bill of rights.* Albany: Public Policy and Education Fund of New York.

Kaplan, M. (1966). *Clinical practice with caregivers of dementia patients.* Bristol, PA: Taylor and Francis.

Keane, P. S. (1993). *Health care reform: A Catholic view.* New York: Paulist.

Keigher, S. M. (1977). What role for social work in the new health care practice paradigm? *Health and Social Work, 22*(2), 149-155.

Keigher, S. M. (1996). Speaking of personal responsibility and individual accountability... *Health and Social Work, 21*(4), 304-311.

Kerson, T. S., et al. (1989). *Social work in health settings: Practice in context.* Binghamton, NY: Haworth.

Kornblum, W., & Smith, C. (1994). *The healing experience: Readings on the social context of health care.* Englewood Cliffs, NJ: Prentice Hall.

Kugelman, W. (1992). Social work ethics in the practice arena: A qualitative study. *Social Work in Health Care, 17*(4), 59-80.

Lassiter, S. M. (1995). *Multicultural clients: A professional handbook for health care providers and social workers.* Westport, CT: Greenwood.

Leutz, W. N., et al. (1985). *Changing health care for an aging society: Planning for the social health maintenance organization.* Lexington, MA: Lexington Books.

Levin, B. L., & Petrila, J. (Eds.). (1996). *Mental health services: A public health perspective.* New York: Oxford University Press.

Lind, R., & Bachman, D. H. (Eds.). (1997). *Fundamentals of perinatal social work: A guide to clinical practice with women, infants, and families.* New York: Haworth, published as a special issue of Social Work and Health Care, 24, 3/4.

Lister, L., & Shore, D. (Eds.). (1984). *Human sexuality in medical social work.* Binghamton, NY: Haworth.

Livingston, I. L. (Ed.). (1994). *Handbook of black American health: The mosaic of conditions, issues, policies, and prospects.* Westport, CT: Greenwood.

Long, D. (1995, June). Attention deficit disorder and case management: Infusing macro social work practice. *Journal of Sociology and Social Welfare,* 45-55.

Lurie, A. (1987). Entrepreneurialism in health care: Implications for social work practice and education. *Journal of Independent Social Work, 2*(1), 7-18.

Lynch, V., & Wilson, P. (Eds.). (1966). *Caring for the HIV/AIDS caregiver.* Westport, CT: Greenwood.

Macklin, R. (1984). Ethical issues in treatment of patients with end-stage renal disease. *Social Work in Health Care, 9*(4), 11-20.

MacLean, M. J., & Sakadakis, V. (1989). Quality of life in terminal care with institutionalized ethnic elderly people. *International Social Work, 32*(3), 209-221.

Mailick, M. D., & Caroff, P. (1996). Professional social work education and health care: Challenges for the future. *Social Work in Health Care, 24*(1/2), 1-7.

Mailick, M. D., & Ullmann, A. (1984). A social work perspective on ethical practice in end-stage renal disease. *Social Work in Health Care., 9*(4), 21-31.

Marcenko, M. O., & Smith, L. K. (1992). The impact of a family-centered case management approach. *Social Work in Health Care, 17*(1), 87-100.

Marcus, L. J. (1990). Research on organizational issues in health care social work. *Social Work in Health Care, 15*(1), 79-95.

Marcyznski-Music, K. K. (1994). *Health care solutions: Designing community-based systems that work.* San Francisco: Jossey-Bass.

Mayer, D., & Vadasey, P. (1966). *Living with a brother or sister with special needs: A book for sibs* (2nd rev. ed.). Seattle: University of Washington Press.

Mayer, J. (1995). The effective healthcare social work director: Managing the social work department at Beth Israel Hospital. *Social Work in Health Care, 20*(4), 61-72.

McCullough, L. B., & Wilson, N. L. (Eds.). (1995). *Long-term care decisions: Ethical and conceptual dimensions.* Baltimore: Johns Hopkins University Press.

McKenzie, N. F. (Ed.). (1994). *Beyond crisis: Confronting health care in the United States.* New York: Meridian.

Miller, J. (1991). *Community based long-term care: Innovative models.* Newbury Park, CA: Sage.

Miller, R. S., & Rehr, H. (1984). *Social work issues in health care.* Englewood Cliffs, NJ: Prentice Hall.

Mizrahi, T. (1992). Social work in health care regulation and legislation. *Health and Social Work, 17*(2), 87-92.

Monk, A. (Ed.). (1990). *Handbook of gerontological services* (2nd ed.). New York: Columbia University Press.

Montague, M. (1993). Geriatric case management as a social work function. Doctoral dissertation, University of Pennsylvania.

Moore, S. (1990, Sept.). A social work practice model of case management: The case management grid. *Social Work*, 444-448.

Morrow-Howell, N. (1992). Clinical case management: The hallmark of gerontological social work. *Journal of Gerontological Social Work*, 18(3/4), 119-131.

Moxley, D. (1996). Teaching case management: Essential content for the preservice preparation of effective personnel. *Journal of Teaching in Social Work*, 13(1/2), 111-140.

Mullaney, J. W., & Andrews, B. F. (1983). Legal problems and principles in discharge planning: Implications for social work. *Social Work in Health Care*, 9(1), 53-62.

Munson, C. (1996, June). Autonomy and managed care in clinical social work practice. *Smith College Studies in Social Work*, 66(3), 241-260.

Netting, F. (1992, March). Case management: Service or symptom? *Social Work*, 160-164.

Netting, F. E., & Williams, F. G. (1996). Case manager-physician collaboration: Implications for professional identity, roles, and relationships. *Health and Social Work*, 21(3), 216-224.

Newton, D. E. (1992). *AIDS issues: A handbook*. Hillside, NJ: Enslow.

Nicholson, J, Young, S. D., Simon, L., Bateman, A., & Fisher, W. H. (1996). Impact of medicaid managed care on child and adolescent emergency mental health screening in Massachusetts. *Psychiatric Services*, 47, 1344-1350.

Nokes, K. M., (Ed.). (1996). *HIV/AIDS and the older adult*. Washington, DC: Hemisphere.

Oktay, J., Steinwachs, D., Mamon, J., Bone, L., & Fahey, M. (1992, November). Evaluating social work discharge planning services for elderly people: Access, complexity, and outcome. *Health and Social Work*, 17(4), 290-298.

Olson, E., Chiclian, E., & Libow, L. (Eds.). (1995). *Controversies in ethics in long-term care*. New York: Springer.

Ory, M. G., & Dunker, A. P. (Eds.). (1992). *In-home care for older people: Health and supportive services*. Newbury Park, CA: Sage.

Oss, M. (1996). Managed behavioral health care: A look at the numbers. *Behavioral Health Management*, 16(3), 16-17.

Oss, M. (1997). Outcome measurement: Work in progress. *Behavioral Health Management*, 17, 4.

Paradis, L. F. (Ed.). (1987). *Stress and burnout among providers caring for the terminally ill and their families*. New York: Haworth.

Parry, J. K. (1989). *Social work theory and practice with the terminally ill*. Binghamton, NY: Haworth.

Pelham, A. O., & Clark, W. F. (Eds.). (1986). *Managing home care for the elderly: Lessons from community-based services*. New York: Springer.

Penney, D. (1997). Friend or foe: The impact of managed care on self-help. *Social Policy*, 27, 48-53.

Perloff, J. D. (1996). Medicaid managed care and urban poor people: Implications for social work. *Health and Social Work*, 21(4), 189-195.

Polinsky, M., Fred, C., & Ganz, P. (1991, August). Quantitative and qualitative assessment of a case management program for cancer patients. *Health and Social Work*, 176-183.

Pollin, I., & Kanean, S. B. (1995). *Medical crisis counseling: Short-term therapy for long-term illness*. New York: Norton.

Poole, D. L. (1996). Keeping managed care in balance. *Health and Social Work*, 21(3), 163-166.

Pray, J. E. (1992). Maximizing the patient's uniqueness and strengths: A challenge for home health care. *Social Work and Health Care*, 17(3), 71-79.

Prichard, E. R., et al. (Eds.). (1977). *Social work with the dying patient and the family.* New York: Columbia University Press.

Reamer, F. G. (Ed.). (1991). *AIDS and ethics.* New York: Columbia University Press.

Reamer, F. G. (1997). Managed ethics under managed care. *Families in Society,* 86-91.

Rehr, H., & Rosenberg, G. (1991). Social health care: Problems and predictions. *Social Work in Health Care, 15*(4), 97-120.

Resnick, C., & Tighe, E. (1997). The role of multidisciplinary community clinics in managed care systems. *Social Work, 42*(1), 91-98.

Rivlin, A. M., & Wiener, J. M. (1988). *Caring for the disabled elderly: Who will pay?* Washington, DC: Brookings Institution.

Rohland, B. M., & Rohrer, J. E. (1996). Best practices: Evaluation of managed mental health care for medicaid enrollees in Iowa. *Psychiatric Services, 47,* 1185-1187.

Rose, S. M. (1992). *Case management and social work practice.* New York: Longman.

Rosenberg, G., & Clarke, S. S. (Eds.). (1987, Spring). Social workers in health care management: The move to leadership. *Social Work in Health Care, 12*(3), entire issue.

Rosenberg, G., & Weissman, A. (Eds.). (1994). *Social work in ambulatory care: New implications for health and social services.* New York: Haworth.

Rothenberg, E. (1994). Bereavement intervention with vulnerable populations: A case report on group work with the developmentally disabled. *Social Work with Groups, 17*(3), 61-75.

Rothman, J. (1992). *Guidelines for case management: Putting research to professional use.* Itasca, IL: F.E. Peacock.

Rothman, J. (1994). *Practice with highly vulnerable clients: Case management and community-based service.* Englewood Cliffs, NJ: Prentice Hall.

Rusnack, B., Schaefer, S. M., & Moxley, D. (1988). "Safe passage": Social work roles and functions in hospice care. *Social Work in Health Care, 13*(3), 3-20.

Rusnack, B., Schaefer, S. M., & Moxley, D. (1990). Hospice: Social work's response to a new form of social caring. *Social Work in Health Care, 15*(2), 95-119.

Ryan, M. (1996, Sept.). Walking in a minefield: Findings from a survey of social workers in Australian hospice and palliative care programs. *Australian Social Work,* 47-54.

Sands, R. C. (1991). *Clinical social work practice in community mental health.* New York: Macmillan.

Sands, R. (1983). Crisis intervention and social work practice in hospitals. *Health and Social Work, 8*(4), 253-261.

Sands, R. G. (1989). The social worker joins the team: A look at the socialization process. *Social Work in Health Care, 14*(2), 1-14.

Sands, R. G., Staffor, J., & McClelland, M. (1990). 'I beg to differ': Conflict in the interdisciplinary team. *Social Work in Health Care, 14*(3), 55-72.

Schmidt, M. G. (1990). *Negotiating a good old age: Challenges of residential living in late life.* San Francisco: Jossey-Bass.

Schmidt, W. H., & Finnegan, J. P. (1993). *TQManager: A practical guide for managing in a total quality organization.* San Francisco: Jossey-Bass.

Schneider, R. L., & Kropf, N. P. (Eds.). (1992). *Gerontological social work knowledge, service settings, and special populations.* Chicago: Nelson-Hall.

Schreiber, H. (1981). Discharge planning: Key to the future of hospital social work. *Health and Social Work, 6*(2), 48-53.

Shapiro, J. (1995). The downside of managed mental health care. *Clinical Social Work Journal, 23*(4), 441-451.

Sheppard, M. (1992, August). Contact and collaboration with general practitioners: A comparison of social workers and community psychiatric nurses. *British Journal of Social Work*, 419-436.

Shera, W. (1996). Managed care and people with severe mental illness: Challenges and opportunities for social work. *Health and Social Work*, *21*(4), 196-201.

Sherman, S. R., & Newman, E. S. (1988). *Foster families for adults: A community alternative in long-term care.* New York: Columbia University Press.

Shipsey, M. (1979). Acute care: A crisis and an opportunity. *Social Work in Health Care*, *5*(1), 19-58.

Siebold, C. (1992). *The hospice movement: Easing death's pains.* New York: Twayne.

Siegel, K. (1990). Psychosocial oncology research. *Social Work in Health Care*, *15*(1), 21-43.

Simmons, J. (1994). Community based care: The new health social work paradigm. *Social Work in Health Care*, *20*(1), 35-46.

Smith, G. C., et al. (Eds.). (1995). *Strengthening aging families: Diversity in practice and policy.* Thousand Oaks, CA: Sage.

Soskis, C. W., & Kerson, T. S. (1992). The Patient Self Determination Act: Opportunity knocks again. *Social Work in Health Care*, *16*(4), 1-18.

Spitzer, W. J., & Nash, K. B. (1996). Educational preparation for contemporary health care social work practice. *Social Work in Health Care*, *24*(1/2), 9-34.

Spitzer, W. J., & Neely, K. (1992). Critical incident stress: The role of hospital based social work in developing a statewide intervention system for first responders delivering emergency services. *Social Work in Health Care*, *18*(1), 39-58.

Springer, D., & Brubaker, T. H. (1984). *Family caregivers and dependent elderly: Minimizing stress and maximizing independence.* Beverly Hills, CA: Sage.

Stine, G. J. (1993). *Acquired immune deficiency syndrome: Biological, medical, social, and legal issues.* Englewood Cliffs, NJ: Prentice Hall.

Strom-Gottfried, K. (1998). Applying a conflict resolution framework to disputes in managed care. *Social Work*, *43*(5), 393-401.

Strom-Gottfried, K. (1997). The implications of managed care for social work education. *Journal of Social Work Education*, *33*(1), pp. 7-18.

Strom-Gottfried, K., & Corcoran, K. (1998). Confronting ethical dilemmas in managed care: Guidelines for students and faculty. *Journal of Social Work Education*, *34*(1), 109-119.

Sunday, R. (1997). Advocacy in the new world of managed care. *Families in Society*, 84-93.

Takahasi, E. A., & Tumbull, J. E. (1994). New findings in psychiatric genetics: Implications for social work practice. *Social Work in Health Care*, *20*(2), 1-21.

Tolson, E. R. (1988). *Metamodel and clinical social work.* New York: Columbia University Press.

Trevillion, S. (1988, April). Conferencing the crisis: The application of network models to social work practice. *British Journal of Social Work*, 289-307.

Turner, F. J. (Ed). (1992). *Mental health and the elderly: Social work perspectives.* New York: Free Press.

Valentine, D. P. (1986). Psychological impact of infertility: Identifying issues and needs. *Social Work in Health Care*, *11*(4), 61-69.

Van Hook, M. P., Berkman, B., & Dunkle, R. (1966). Assessment tools for general health care settings: PRIME-AID, OARS, and SF-36. *Health and Social Work*, *21*(4), 230-234.

Volland, P. (1996). Social work practice in health care: Looking to the future with a different lens. *Social Work in Health Care*, *24*(1/2), 35-51.

Vourlekis, B. S., & Greene, R. (Eds.). (1992). *Social work case management.* New York: Aldine de Gruyter.

Vourlekis, B. S., Bakke-Friedland, K., & Zlotnik, J. L. (1995). Clinical indicators to assess the quality of social work services in nursing homes. *Social Work in Health Care, 22*(1), 81-93.

Vourlekis, B. S., Greene, R. R., Gelfand, D. E., & Zlotnik, J. L. (1992). Searching for the doable in nursing home social work practice. *Social Work in Health Care, 17*(3), 45-70.

Wallace, H. (1996). *Family violence: Legal, medical, and social perspectives.* Boston: Allyn and Bacon.

Walther, V. N. (1990). Emerging roles of social work in perinatal services. *Social Work in Health Care, 15*(2), 35-48.

Watt, W. J., & Kallman, G. L. (1998). Managing professional obligations under managed care: A social work perspective. *Family Community Health, 21*(2), 41-49.

Wennberg, J. E. (1990). Outcomes research, cost containment, and the fear of health care rationing. *New England Journal of Medicine, 323*(20).

Wesley, C. A. (1996). Social work and end-of-life decisions: Self-determination and the common good. *Health and Social Work, 21*(2), 115-121.

White, J. (1995). *Competing solutions: American health care proposals and international experience.* Washington, DC: Brookings Institution.

Winegar, N. (1993). Managed mental health care: Implications for administrators and managers of community-based agencies. *Families in Society,* 171-177.

Wisby, M., Rosendale, E., & Gorbien, M. (1996). The family meeting: A benchmark of high-quality geriatric care. *Continuum, 16*(5), 10-17.

Wood, D. (Ed.). (1992). *Delivering health care to homeless persons: The diagnosis and management of medical and mental health conditions.* New York: Springer.

Worden, J. (1966). *The grieving child: When a parent dies.* New York: Guilford.

York, G. Y. (1987). Religious-based denial in the NICU: Implications for social work. *Social Work in Health Care, 12*(4), 31-45.

State University of New York, University at Albany
School of Social Welfare

Course Title: Social Work Practice in Health Care Settings (R SSW 749-5947)
Fall 1996

Course Instructor: Julie Abramson

DESCRIPTION

This course will focus on the development of social work practice skills relevant to health care settings, including assessment of the impact of illness, disability, treatment and hospitalization on patients and families; the phases of the helping process will be reviewed for specific application in health care settings and appropriate theoretical models for practice identified and applied to practice situations, particularly those related to discharge planning, chronic and terminal illness, family conflict and resource development. Consideration will be given to the effects of class, race, gender, sexual orientation, culture and ethnicity on practice with various populations and problems in health care settings.

In addition, the policy, organizational and ethical context of social work practice in health care will be considered as will interdisciplinary issues and sources of interdisciplinary strain. Socialization processes will be examined with emphasis on strategies for working with other professionals, particularly physicians and nurses. Skills in teamwork, program development and work with groups will be emphasized.

OBJECTIVES

1. To integrate knowledge of the meaning of illness, disability and loss for patients and families with general clinical understanding of human behavior and the life cycle to form a base for social work practice in health care settings.

2. To learn about the role of social class, race, gender, sexual orientation, culture and ethnicity in affecting health behavior and adaptation to illness, disability and loss, and to understand the implications of this information for social work practice in health care settings; to strive for awareness of the impact of illness, class, race, gender, sexual orientation, culture and ethnicity on oneself in the process of working with patients and families in health care settings.

3. To understand and selectively utilize those theoretical models of social work practice most appropriate to practice in health care settings, in particular, crisis theory, the life model or ecological approaches, family systems and task-centered treatment; to base choice of practice model on available knowledge regarding outcome with particular populations and problems.

4. To learn strategies of engagement, assessment, contracting and intervention most relevant to situations that arise with clients and families in health care settings, in particular: discharge planning, terminal and chronic illness, decision making, family conflict and long-term care.

5. To identify key issues in interdisciplinary collaboration and teamwork and to use this understanding in developing strategic interventions with other professionals and teams.

6. To understand the policy, organizational and ethical context of social work practice in health care; to identify needed changes in policy at a macro and organizational level in order to make a better fit between client and practice realities and policy.

TEXTS

There is no required text. A readings packet will cover the course content and will be available on reserve.

Recommended Texts

S. Shem. (1978). *The house of God.* New York: Dell.

EVALUATION

The class will follow a seminar format interspersed with lectures. Class participation, based on assigned readings, will receive particular emphasis, especially in light of small class size. Therefore staying current with reading assignments will be expected, as will regular attendance.

Students are expected to complete the following assignments:

1. Log on Integration of Readings with Practice - Entries Due on Sessions 4, 8, and 13.

A readings log is to be prepared based on a selection of 8 readings from the syllabus (you can include recommended readings) that seem most relevant to your current practice setting; a critical analysis of its relevance to practice and actual or possible applications to practice in the student's placement setting will be the focus of the log entry, although specific points from the readings should be alluded to. Each reading should be selected from a different week's assignment, unless you ask the instructor for permission to read more than one article assigned for the same session. This assignment will account for 20% of the final grade.

2. Midterm Assessment Paper - Due Session 7.

A paper not to exceed 15 pages on assessment of and intervention with a client system in a health care setting will be due on and will account for 45% of the final grade. The assignment outline will be handed out shortly after the beginning of the semester. For those students not in health settings, it is possible to do a research paper on a particular issue in social work practice in health care, with particular emphasis on practice concerns. You will need to discuss this with me.

3. Analysis of a Process Recording of a Collaborative Contact - Due Session 14.

A paper not to exceed 3-5 pages (excluding the process recording) that analyzes a collaborative contact with another health care professional or with a community agency contact person. The contact should be selected based on the complexity or difficulty in handling the particular collaborative exchange. This paper will account for 20% of the grade.

4. Class Participation

Evaluation of class participation will count for 15% of the grade and will reflect participation in sharing a case with the class as well as general contribution to class discussion.

All papers are to be typed (except for actual process recordings which may be handwritten), double spaced and carefully checked for typographical and spelling errors (reference lists should be single spaced). Use APA style for citing references in the paper and in compiling the reference list. If inadequate attention is paid to writing (grammar, spelling and typos) and presentation of the paper, the paper grade will be reduced, as it will if it is late without satisfactory explanation prior to due date. Plagiarism will result in a failing evaluation for the course as will any other form of cheating. Students are strongly encouraged to complete all assigned work during the semester. Incompletes must be requested and will be granted only in extraordinary circumstances. Any incompletes must be removed by the end of the following semester or a failing grade will result.

COURSE OUTLINE

All readings listed below are required and are to be completed prior to the class date for which they are assigned (with the exception of those for the first class).

Session 1. The Context of Social Work Practice in Health Care
Course overview
History
Social work role & function
Medical model
Policy issues

Readings
J. Ross. (1995). Hospital social work. In. R.L. Edwards (Ed.-in-Chief), *Encyclopedia of social work* (19th ed.) (pp. 1365-1376). Washington, DC: NASW Press.

P. Klass. (1987). Camels, zebras, and fascinomas, 67-71, and Curing, 200-205. *A not entirely benign procedure.* New York: G.P. Putnam.

C. Berger, J. Cayner, G. Jensen, T. Mizrahi, A. Scesny, & J. Trachtenberg. (1996). The changing scene of social work in hospitals: A report of a national study by the Society for Social Work Administrators in Health Care and NASW. *Health and Social Work, 21*(3), 167-177.

J.S. Abramson. (1993). Orienting social work employees in interdisciplinary settings: Shaping professional and organizational perspectives. *Social Work, 38*(2), 152-157.

J.S. Abramson. (1992). Health-related problems. In W.J. Reid (Ed.), *Task strategies: An empirical approach to clinical social work* (pp. 223-247). New York: Columbia University Press.

Recommended
S. Busca. (1994). Insights about social work field placements in a teaching hospital: Preparation for generalist practice. In M. Holosko & P. Taylor (Eds.), *Social work practice in health care settings* (pp. 33-41). Toronto: Canadian Scholars' Press.

F. Reamer. (1992). Facing up to the challenge of diagnosis related groups. In S. Rose (Ed.), *Case management in social work practice* (pp. 135-148). White Plains, NY: Longman.

B. Harper. (1990). Blacks and the health care delivery system: Challenges and prospects. In S. Logan, E. Freeman, & R. McRoy (Eds.), *Social work practice with black families* (pp. 239-256). White Plains, NY: Longman.

Session 2. Impact of Illness and Hospitalization on Patients and Families
Readings
J. Rolland. (1994). The psychosocial typology of illness. In *Families, illness and disability: An integrative treatment model* (pp. 20-42). New York: Basic Books.

J. Rolland. (1994). The time phases of illness. In *Families, illness and disability: An integrative treatment model* (pp. 42-59). New York: Basic Books.

R. Kotlowitz. (1994, Dec. 4). From my wife's room. *New York Times Magazine.* (class handout).

J. Ross. (1993). Understanding the family experience with childhood cancer. In N. Stearns, M. Lauria, J. Hermann, & P. Fogelberg (Eds.), *Oncology social work: A clinician's guide* (pp. 199-236). Atlanta, GA: American Cancer Society.

Recommended

R.H. Moos & J. Schaeffer. (1984). The crisis of physical illness. In R.H. Moos (Ed.), *Coping with physical illness: A second perspective* (pp. 3-25). New York: Plenum.

K. Ell & H. Northen. (1990). Research on health, illness & family. In K. Ell & H. Northen, *Families & health care: Psychosocial practice* (pp. 25-54). Hawthorne, NY: Aldine de Gruyter.

T. Kerson. (1985). *Understanding chronic illness: The medical and psychosocial dimensions of nine diseases.* New York: Free Press.

T. Kerson. (1989). *Social work in health settings: Practice in context.* Binghamton, NY: Haworth.

J. Interrante. (1986). To have without holding: Memories of life with a person with AIDS. In M. Witt (Ed.), *AIDS and patient management: Legal, cultural and social issues* (pp. 121-124). Owings Mills, MD: Rynd Communications.

M. Mailick. (1979). The impact of severe illness on the individual and the family: An overview. *Social Work in Health Care, 5*(2), 117-128.

N. Stearns, M. Lauria, J. Hermann, & P. Fogelberg (Eds.). (1993). *Oncology social work: A clinician's guide.* Atlanta, GA: American Cancer Society.

Session 3. Impact of Culture & Ethnicity

Readings

Everyone should read the next four readings; use the recommended readings where they are relevant to your interests or caseload.

A. Harwood. (1981). Guidelines for culturally appropriate health care. In A. Harwood (Ed), *Ethnicity and medical care*, 3rd. ed. (pp. 482-507). Cambridge: Harvard University Press.

R. Maduro. (1983). Curanderismo and Latino views of disease and curing. *Western Journal of Medicine, 139*, 868-870.

S. Logan, E. Freeman, & R. McRoy. (1990). Treatment considerations for working with pregnant Black adolescents, their families and their partners. In S. Logan, E. Freeman & R. McRoy (Eds.), *Social work practice with Black families* (pp. 148-168). White Plains, NY: Longman.

E. Congress. (1992). Cultural differences in health beliefs: Implications for social work practice in health care settings. *Social Work in Health Care, 17*(3), 81-93.

Recommended

J. Hartog & A. Hartog. (1983). Cultural aspects of health and illness behavior in hospitals. *Western Journal of Medicine, 139*(6), 106-112.

N. Scheper-Hughes & D. Stewart. (1983). Curanderismo in Taos County, NM—A possible case of anthropological romanticism? *Western Journal of Medicine, 139*, 875-884.

A. Walker. (1990). Beauty: When the other dancer is the self. In E. White (Ed.), *The Black woman's health book* (pp. 280-287). Seattle, WA: Seal Press.

G. Arnold. (1990). Coming home: One Black woman's journey to health and fitness. In E. White (Ed.), *The Black woman's health book* (pp. 269-279). Seattle, WA: Seal Press.

M. Lai & K.K. Yue. (1990). The Chinese. In N.W. Morrison, J. Anderson, & E. Richards (Eds.), *Cross-cultural caring* (pp. 68-90). Vancouver, Canada: University of British Columbia Press.

J. Glasgow & E. Adaskin. (1990). The West Indians. In N.W. Morrison, J. Anderson, & E. Richards (Eds.), *Cross-cultural caring* (pp. 214-244). Vancouver, Canada: University of British Columbia Press.

D. Gleave & A. Manes. (1990). The Central Americans. In N.W. Morrison, J. Anderson & E. Richards (Eds.), *Cross-cultural caring* (pp. 36-67). Vancouver, Canada: University of British Columbia Press.

T. LaFromboise. (1988). American Indian mental health policy. *American Psychologist, 43*(5), 388-397.

S. Mercer. (1996). Navajo elderly people in a reservation nursing home: Admission predictors and culture care practices. *Social Work, 41*(2), 181-189.

Session 4. Assessment & Intervention Depression
Readings
C. Germain. (1984). The professional frame of reference as context for practice. In C. Germain, *Social work practice in health care: An ecological perspective* (pp. 57-86). New York: Free Press.

C. Cowger. (1992). Assessment of client strengths. In D. Saleebey (Ed.), *The strengths perspective in social work practice*, 2nd ed. (pp. 139-147). New York: Longman. [Just review list of possible client strengths.]

M. Wool. (1990). Understanding depression in medical patients, Part I: Diagnostic considerations. *Social Work in Health Care, 14*(4), 25-38.

M. Wool. (1990). Understanding depression in medical patients, Part II: Clinical intervention. *Social Work in Health Care, 14*(4), 38-52.

Recommended
M. Mailick. (1990). The short-term treatment of depression of physically ill hospital patients. In K. Davidson & S. Clarke (Eds.), *Social work in health care: A handbook for practice* (Part 1, pp. 401-414). Binghamton, NY: Haworth.

J. Wood Wetzel. (1994). Depression: Women at risk. *Social Work in Health Care, 19*(3/4), 85-108.

Session 5. Family Assessment & Intervention Dementia
Readings
S. McDaniel, J. Hepworth, & W. Doherty. (1993). A new prescription for family health care. *The Networker, 17*(1), 19-63.

D. Monahan. (1993). Assessment of dementia patients and their families: An ecological-family-centered approach. *Health and Social Work, 18*(2), 123-130.

F. Gibson. (1993). Use of the past. In. A. Chapman & M. Marshall (Eds.), *Dementia: New skills for social workers* (pp. 40-62). London: Jessica Kingsley.

J. Sherlock & I. Gardner. (1993). Systemic family intervention. In. A. Chapman & M. Marshall (Eds.), *Dementia: New skills for social workers* (pp. 63-79). London: Jessica Kingsley.

Recommended
K. Ell & H. Northen. (1990). *Families and health care: Psychosocial practice.* White Plains, NY: Aldine de Gruyter. (Chapter 7, Family Therapy, pp. 155-171; skim earlier part of chapter for relevant material.)

Session 6. Family Assessment & Intervention II

Readings
S. Gonzalez, P. Steinglass, & D. Reiss. (1989). Putting the illness in its place: Discussion groups for families with chronic medical illnesses. *Family Process, 28*, 69-87.

J.S. Abramson, J. Donnelly, M. King, & M. Mailick. (1993). Disagreements in discharge planning: A normative phenomenon. *Health and Social Work, 18*(1), 57-64.

C. Cox & A. Monk. (1993). Hispanic culture and family care of Alzheimer's patients. *Health and Social Work, 18*(2), 92-100.

M. Perez & C. Pilsecker. (1990). Family therapy with spinal cord injured substance abusers. *Social Work in Health Care, 14*(2), 15-25.

Recommended

L. Videka-Sherman. (1991). Child abuse & neglect. In A. Gitterman (Ed.), *Handbook of social work practice with vulnerable populations* (pp. 345-381). New York: Columbia University Press.

B. Carlson. (1991). Domestic violence. In A. Gitterman (Ed.), *Handbook of social work practice with vulnerable populations* (pp. 471-502). New York: Columbia University Press.

J. Hirschwald. (1989). Rehabilitation of a quadriplegic adolescent; Regional spinal cord injury center. In T. Kerson (Ed.), *Social work in health settings: Practice in context* (pp. 157-176). Binghamton, NY: Haworth.

Session 7. Terminal Illness
Advance Directives

Readings

M. Glajchen, D. Blum, & K. Calder. (1995). Cancer pain management and the role of social work: Barriers and interventions. *Health and Social Work, 20*(3), 200-206.

G. Christ. (1993). Psychosocial tasks throughout the cancer experience. In N. Stearns, M. Lauria, J. Hermann, & P. Fogelberg (Eds.), *Oncology social work: A clinician's guide* (pp. 79-99). Atlanta, GA: American Cancer Society.

M. Freedman. (1994). Helping home bound elderly clients understand and use advance directives. *Social Work in Health Care, 20*(2), 61-73).

K. Wilber & S. Reynolds. (1995). Rethinking alternatives to guardianship. *The Gerontologist, 35*(2), 248-257.

C. Soskis & T. Kerson. (1992). The patient self-determination act: Opportunity knocks again. *Social Work in Health Care, 16*(4), 1-18.

Recommended

M. Mailick. (1984). Lost opportunity: Terminal illness in middle age. In L. Suszycki, et al. (Eds.), *Social work and terminal care* (pp. 31-41). New York: Praeger.

J. Hinton. (1984). Coping with terminal illness. In R. Fitzpatrick et al. (Eds.), *The experience of illness* (pp. 226-245). London: Tavistock.

K. Orloff Kaplan. (1995). End of life decisions. In R.L. Edwards (Ed.-in-Chief), *Encyclopedia of social work.* (19th ed., pp. 857-868). Washington, DC: NASW Press.

A. Hanlan. (1984). Notes of a dying professor. In T. Carlton (Ed.), *Clinical social work in health settings* (pp. 245-258). New York: Springer

N. Millet Fish. (1989). Hospice: Terminal Illness, teamwork and the quality of life. In T. Kerson (Ed.), *Social work in health settings: Practice in context* (pp. 449-469). Binghamton, NY: Haworth.

N. Stearns, M. Lauria, J. Hermann, & P. Fogelberg (Eds.). (1993). *Oncology social work: A clinician's guide.* Atlanta, GA: American Cancer Society.

Session 8. Discharge Planning & Models of Intervention

Readings

E. Simon, N. Showers, S. Blumenfield, G. Holden, & X. Wu. (1995). Delivery of home care services after discharge: What really happens. *Health and Social Work, 20*(1), 5-14.

J. S. Abramson. (1989). Enhancing patient participation: Clinical strategies in the discharge planning process. *Social Work in Health Care, 14*(4), 53-71.

C. Bennett, J. Legon, & F. Zilberfein. (1989). The significance of empathy in current hospital based practice. *Social Work in Health Care, 14*(2), 27-41.

E. Proctor, N. Morrow-Howell, & C. Lott. (1993). Classification & correlates of ethical dilemmas in hospital social work. *Social Work, 38*(2), 166-177.

Recommended

F. Nason. (1990). Beyond relationship: The current challenge in clinical practice. *Social Work in Health Care, 14*(4), 9-24.

C. James. (1987). An ecological approach to defining discharge planning in social work. *Social Work in Health Care, 12*(4), 47-59.

M. Hunt & G. Hunt. (1983). Simulated site visits in the relocation of older people. *Health and Social Work, 8*(1), 5-14.

S. Mercer & R. Kane. (1979). Helplessness and hopelessness among the institutionalized aged: An experiment. *Health and Social Work, 4*(1), 91-115.

E. Langer & J. Rodin. (1976). The effects of choice and enhanced personal responsibility for the aged. *Journal of Personality and Social Psychology, 34*, 191-198.

J. Abramson. (1988). Participation of elderly patients in discharge planning: Is self determination a reality? *Social Work, 33*(5), 443-448.

J. Feather. (1993). Factors in perceived hospital discharge planning effectiveness. *Social Work in Health Care, 19*(1), 1-14.

T. Kerson & J. Zelinka. (1989). Discharge planning: Acute medical services. In T. Kerson, *Social work in health settings: Practice in context* (pp. 195-214). Binghamton, NY: Haworth.

Session 9. AIDS

Readings

S. Jue. (1994). Psychosocial issues of AIDS long term survivors. *Families in Society, 75*(6), 324-332.

H. Land. (1994). AIDS and women of color. *Families in Society, 75*(6), 355-361.

S. Taylor-Brown. (1995). HIV/AIDS: Direct practice. In R.L. Edwards (Ed.-in-Chief), *Encyclopedia of social work* (19th ed., pp. 1291-1314). Washington, DC: NASW Press.

P. Haney. (1988). Providing empowerment to the person with AIDS. *Social Work, 33*(3), 251-253.

Recommended

Families in Society, 75(6)-HIV/AIDS, A Special Issue. (Entire issue)

R. Weitz. (1990). Uncertainty and the lives of persons with AIDS. In P. Conrad & R. Kerns (Eds.), *The sociology of health and illness: Critical perspectives* (3rd ed., pp. 111-122). New York: St. Martin's.

B. Dicks. (1994). African American Women and AIDS: A public health/social work challenge. *Social Work in Health Care, 19*(3/4), 123-143.

G. Lloyd. (1995). HIV/AIDS overview. In R.L. Edwards (Ed.-in-Chief), *Encyclopedia of social work* (19th ed., pp. 1257-1290). Washington, DC: NASW Press.

K. J. Peterson. (1995). HIV/AIDS: Women. In R.L. Edwards (Ed.-in-Chief), *Encyclopedia of social work* (19th ed., pp. 1325-1330). Washington, DC: NASW Press.

L. Wiener, C. DeVane Fair, & A. Garcia. (1995). HIV/AIDS: Pediatric. In R.L. Edwards (Ed.-in-Chief), *Encyclopedia of social work* (19th ed., pp. 1314-1324). Washington, DC: NASW Press.

Session 10. Primary and Community-based Care
Readings

G. Rosenberg. (1994). Social work, the family and the community. *Social Work in Health Care, 20*(1), 7-20.

S. Logan, E. Freeman, & R. McRoy. (1990). Treatment considerations for working with pregnant Black adolescents, their families and their partners. In. S. Logan, E. Freeman, & R. McRoy (Eds.), *Social work practice with Black families* (pp. 148-168). White Plains, NY: Longman.

J. Oktay. (1995). *Primary health care.* In R.L. Edwards (Ed.-in-Chief), *Encyclopedia of social work* (19th. ed., pp. 1887-1894). Washington, DC: NASW Press.

J. Simmons. (1994). Community based care: The new health social work paradigm. *Social Work in Health Care, 20*(1), 35-46.

D. Keehn, C. Roglitz, & M.L. Bowden (1994). Impact of social work on recidivism and non-medical complaints in the emergency department. *Social Work in Health Care, 20*(1), 65-74.

P. Wells. (1993). Preparing for sudden death: Social work in the emergency room. *Social Work, 38*(3), 339-342.

Session 11. Long-Term Care
Readings

R. W. Michelsen. (1989). Hospital based case management for the frail elderly. In T. Kerson (Ed.), *Social work in health settings: Practice in context* (pp. 431-448). Binghamton, NY: Haworth.

S. Foldes. (1990). Life in an institution: A sociological and anthropological view. In. R. Kane & A. Caplan (Eds.), *Everyday ethics: Resolving dilemmas in nursing home life* (pp. 21-36). New York: Springer.

R. Kane. (1990). Everyday life in nursing homes. In. R. Kane & A. Caplan (Eds.), *Everyday ethics: Resolving dilemmas in nursing home life* (pp. 3-20). New York: Springer.

R. Kane, A. Caplan, I. Freeman, M. Aroskar, & E. Urv-Wong. (1990). Avenues to appropriate autonomy: What next? In. R. Kane & A. Caplan (Eds.), *Everyday ethics: Resolving dilemmas in nursing home life* (pp. 306-317). New York: Springer.

Recommended

R. Kane & A. Caplan. (Eds.). (1990). *Everyday ethics: Resolving dilemmas in nursing home life.* New York: Springer.

B. Collopy. (1992). Autonomy in long term care: Some crucial distinctions. In. S. Rose (Ed.), *Case management in social work practice* (pp. 56-71). White Plains, NY: Longman.

Session 12. Interdisciplinary Collaboration
Readings

R. Fox. (1980). *The human condition of health professionals.* Durham, NH: Distinguished Lecturer Series, University of New Hampshire.

J. Abramson & T. Mizrahi. (1986). Strategies for enhancing collaboration between social workers and physicians. *Social Work in Health Care, 12*(1), 1-21.

J.S. Abramson & T. Mizrahi. (1996). When social workers and physicians collaborate: Positive and negative interdisciplinary experiences. *Social Work, 41*(3), 270-281.

P. Klass. (1987). Crying in the hospital, 64-66. Macho, 76-84. Learning the language, 72-83. A weekend in the life, 221-245. In *A not entirely benign procedure.* New York: G.P. Putnam.

M. Egan & G. Kadushin. (1995). Competitive allies: Rural nurses' and social workers' perceptions of the social work role in the hospital setting. *Social Work in Health Care, 20*(3), 1-23.

F.E. Netting & F. Williams. (1996). Case manager–physician collaboration: Implications for professional identity, roles and relationships. *Health and Social Work, 21*(3), 216-224.

Recommended

S. Shem. (1978). *The house of God.* NY: Dell.

B. Dana. (1983). The collaborative process. in R. Miller & H. Rehr (Eds.), *Social work issues in health care.* Englewood Cliffs, NJ: Prentice Hall, 181-220.

T. Mizrahi & J. Abramson. (1985). Sources of strain between physicians and social workers: Implications for social workers in health care. *Social Work in Health Care, 10*(3), 33-51.

Session 13. Teamwork

Readings

J. Abramson. (1989). Making teams work. *Social Work with Groups, 12*(4), 45-63.

R. Sands, J. Stafford, & M. McClelland. (1990). I beg to differ: Conflict in the interdisciplinary team. *Social Work in Health Care, 14*(3), 55-72.

T. Drinka & J. Streim. (1994). Case studies from purgatory: Maladaptive behavior within geriatrics health care teams. *The Gerontologist, 34*(4), 541-547.

Recommended

D. Banta & R. Fox. (1972). Role strains of a health care team in a poverty community. *Social Science and Medicine, 6,* 697-722.

Session 14. Current Trends in Social Work in Health Care
Self directed work teams
Restructuring and re-engineering hospitals
Managed care
Community based and continuums of care

Readings

In addition to the following readings, review several articles in the "TRENDS" folder on reserve that cover various trends in the current health care scene.

G. Rosenberg & A. Weissman. (1995). Preliminary thoughts on sustaining central social work departments. *Social Work in Health Care, 20*(4), 111-116.

G. Edinburg & J. Cottler. (1995). Managed care. In R. L. Edwards (Ed.-in-Chief), *Encyclopedia of social work* (19th ed., pp. 1635-1642). Washington, DC: NASW Press.

J. Globerman, J. MacKenzie Davies, & S. Walsh. (1996). Social work in restructuring hospitals: Meeting the challenge. *Health and Social Work, 21*(3), 178-188.

D. Poole. (1996). Keeping managed care in balance. *Health and Social Work, 21*(3), 163-166.

State University of New York, University at Albany
School of Social Welfare

Course Title: Poverty, Health, and Health Policy (RSSW 732)
Spring 1998

Course Instructor: Janet D. Perloff

PURPOSE

This course examines health policies with particular attention to their effects on the poor and other disadvantaged and at-risk populations. In both an historical and a contemporary context, health policies and programs are examined in terms of (1) their underlying assumptions and values; (2) their formulation, development, and implementation; and (3) their effectiveness. Inequalities in health status and access to health care are considered and issues of social and economic justice, discrimination, and oppression are highlighted. Roles played by social workers in addressing the health problems of vulnerable populations are explored and implications of health policies for practice and management are assessed. Consideration is given to alternative policy approaches for addressing the health problems of the poor and other disadvantaged and at-risk populations.

OBJECTIVES

At the conclusion of the course, students are expected to have achieved the following:

1. An understanding of the significance of social, psychological, behavioral, cultural, economic, and political factors in relation to health status and access to health care.

2. An awareness of the influence that assumptions about the determinants of health status and access have on policy formulation, development, implementation, and effectiveness.

3. General familiarity with the content of health policies and programs targeted to meet the needs of the poor, minorities, the elderly, the disabled, and other at-risk populations.

4. An understanding of the implications of health policies for social work practice in health care and other settings and for management of programs and agencies addressing health and related social problems.

5. The ability to analyze critically specific health policies and their implications for social work practice, including concerns for issues of social and economic justice, discrimination, and oppression.

6. An understanding of the health policymaking process.

TEXTS

Along with required journal articles and papers, the following books and reports serve as the main texts for this course:

Abraham, L. K. *Mama Might Be Better Off Dead: The Failure of Health Care in Urban America.* Chicago: The University of Chicago Press, 1993.

Gilbert, N., Specht, H., & Terrell, P. *Dimensions of Social Welfare Policy*, 3rd ed. Englewood Cliffs, NJ: Prentice Hall, 1993.

Longest, B. B. *Health Policymaking in the United States*. Ann Arbor, MI: Health Administration Press, 1994.

Students are also encouraged to visit the Graduate Library, where they can obtain the following:

Brustman, M. J. (1996). *Health Policy: A Guide to Selected Reference Sources*. Unpublished manuscript, University Libraries, State University of New York, University at Albany.

All assigned readings are required and are to be completed prior to the class for which they are assigned. Additional reading may be assigned during the semester. From time to time, newspaper and magazine articles will be assigned by the instructor and these will be the topic of subsequent class discussion.

EVALUATION

The class will follow a lecture-discussion format. All students are expected to (1) prepare for class by reading and thinking about assigned material; (2) attend class; and (3) participate actively in class discussion.

Students are also expected to complete the following assignments:

1. A midterm exam. The midterm will constitute 30% of the final grade.
2. A final exam. The final will constitute 40% of your grade.
3. A 10-page essay analyzing the health policy context of one of the main characters described in Abraham's *Mama Might Be Better Off Dead*. (See Appendix for details.) A recommended schedule for reading this book is provided in the syllabus and a detailed assignment for the final essay will be distributed.

Criteria to be used to grade your essay include the following: (1) research skills (use of library, sources); (2) analytical skills (logical, objective development); (3) integration of course concepts and readings; (4) expressive quality (writing, editing, ease of reading); and (5) insight and innovation (originality, creativity).

This essay constitutes 30% of the final grade and is due at the beginning of the last class. Papers are to be typed, double-spaced, and written in appropriate academic style.

Students are strongly encouraged to complete all assigned work during the semester. Incompletes must be requested and will be granted only in extraordinary circumstances.

OUTLINE

Session	Topic	Session	Topic
1	Introduction	8	Framework for Policy Analysis
2	Determinants of Health	9	Policies Targeting Specific Health Problems of the Poor: Categorical Programs and Block Grants in Health
3	Determinants of Access to Health Care		
4	Policymaking in Health	10	Policies Financing Health Care for the Poor: Medicaid
5	Policymaking in Health		
6	Midterm Exam	11	Medicaid Managed Care
7	Framework for Policy Analysis	12	Final Exam

SCHEDULE

Session 1   Introduction
Introduction to the course
Overview of the policymaking process
Social work roles in the policymaking process

Required Reading
Gilbert, Specht, and Terrell, Chapter 1, The Field of Social Welfare Policy

Session 2   Determinants of Health
Social, biological, behavioral, cultural, environmental, and economic determinants of health
Social inequalities and health: income, race, ethnicity, gender, socioeconomic status
The influence of values and theories about health status determinants on policy choices
Health status of the poor

Required Reading
Longest, Chapter 1

Evans, R. G., & Stoddart, G. L. "Producing Health, Consuming Health Care." In Evans, R. G., Barer, M. L., & Marmor, T. R. (Eds.), *Why Are Some People Healthy and Others Not? The Determinants of Health of Populations.* New York: Aldine de Gruyter, 1994.

Mendoza, F. S. 1994. "The Health of Latino Children in the United States." *The Future of Children,* 4(3): 43-72.

Abraham, Intro, Chapters 1 and 2

Session 3   Determinants of Access to Health Care
Social, behavioral, cultural, and economic determinants of health care access
Access inequalities: The role of income, race, ethnicity, gender, socioeconomic status
The influence of values and theories about access on policy choices
Health care access and the poor
Access to what? Inequalities in access to high-quality care

Required Reading
Andersen, R. 1995. "Revisiting the Behavioral Model and Access to Medical Care: Does It Matter?" *Journal of Health and Social Behavior,* 36(March): 1-10.

Fox, S. A., & Stein, J. A. 1991. "The Effect of Physician-Patient Communication on Mammography Utilization by Different Ethnic Groups." *Medical Care,* 29(11): 1065-1082.

Perloff, J., & Jaffee, K. (in press). "Late Entry Into Prenatal Care: The Neighborhood Context." *Social Work.*

Weinick, R. M., Zuvekas, S. H., & Drilea, S. K. *Access to Health Care — Sources and Barriers, 1996.* (MEPS Research Findings #3. AHCPR Publication No. 98-0001.) Rockville, MD: Agency for Health Care Policy and Research, October 1997.

Abraham, Chapters 3 and 4

Session 4   Policymaking in Health
Overview of the health policymaking process
The political marketplace
Policy formulation — agenda setting and the development of legislation
Social work role in agenda setting

Required Reading
Longest, Chapters 2, 3, 4
Abraham, Chapters 5, 6, 7

Session 5   Policymaking in Health
Policy implementation and modification
Social work role in implementation and modification
Interest groups in health
Social work as an interest group — roles, strategies
Strategies used to influence the policymaking process

Required Reading
Longest, Chapters 5, 6, 7
Abraham, Chapters 8, 9, 10

Session 6   Midterm Exam

Session 7   Framework for Analysis of Health Policy
Theories, assumptions, and values — revisited
Overview of dimensions of health policy choice
Basis of social allocations: Eligibility
Nature of social provisions: Benefits

Required Reading
Gilbert, Specht, & Terrell, Chapter 2, "A Framework for Social Welfare Policy Analysis"; Chapter
    3, "Basis of Social Allocations"; Chapter 4, "Nature of Social Provisions"
Abraham, Chapters 11 and 12

Session 8   Framework for Analysis of Health Policy
Structure of the delivery system
Financing: Sources of funds and systems of transfer

Required Reading
Gilbert, Specht, & Terrell, Chapter 5, "The Structure of the Delivery System"; Chapter 6,
    "Sources of Funds"; Chapter 7, "Systems of Transfer"
Abraham, Chapters 14, 15, Epilogue

**Session 9   Policies Targeted to Specific Health Problems of the Poor: Categorical Programs and
                     Block Grants in Health**
Title V Maternal and Child Health Block Grants and other categorical programs in health

History

Social work role

Analysis of values, assumptions, and policy choices

Required Reading

Andrews, C. *Promoting the Health of Women and Children Through Title V.* Washington, DC: National Governor's Association: June 1995.

Klerman, L. *Alive and Well? A Research and Policy Review of Health Programs for Poor Young Children.* New York: National Center for Children in Poverty, 1991. Chapter 2, " The History of Health Services for Children in Poverty"; Chapter 7, "Programs that Have Improved the Health of Children in Poverty."

Siefert, K. 1983. "An Exemplar of Primary Prevention in Social Work: The Sheppard-Towner Act of 1921." *Social Work in Health Care,* 9(1): 87-103.

Session 10   Policies Financing Health Care For the Poor: Medicaid

History and current status of Medicaid

Analysis of Medicaid policy choices

Key policy issues: access, quality, costs

Implications of choices and issues for clients, social workers, and agencies serving the poor

Required Reading

Longest, Chapter 1, pages 24 and 25 (review)

Physician Payment Review Commission. *Medicaid: Spending Trends and the Move to Managed Care.* Washington, DC: Author. 1997. Chapter 20, "PPRC Annual Report to Congress."

Session 11   Medicaid Managed Care

What is managed care?

History of managed care in health and Medicaid

The Balanced Budget Act of 1997 — Implications

Policy choices associated with Medicaid managed care

Implications of Medicaid managed care for clients, social workers, and agencies serving the poor

Required Reading

Perloff, J. 1996. "Medicaid Managed Care and Urban Poor People: Implications for Social Work." *Health and Social Work,* 21(3):189-195

Sisk, J. E., Gorman, S. A., Reisinger, A. L., Giled, S. A., DuMouchel, W. H., & Hynes, M. M. 1996. "Evaluation of Medicaid Managed Care: Satisfaction, Access, and Use." *Journal of the American Medical Association,* 276: 50-55.

Ware, J. E., Bayliss, M. S., Rogers, W. H., Kosinski, M., & Tarlov, A. R. 1996. "Differences in 4-Year Health Outcomes for Elderly and Poor, Chronically, Ill Patients Treated in HMO and Fee-for-Service Systems." *Journal of the American Medical Association,* 276: 1039-1047.

Session 12   Final Exam

Final Essay Due

APPENDIX

Final Essay Assignment

The goal of this assignment is to give you an opportunity to review the material covered in this course, to demonstrate your mastery of this material, and to apply what you've learned.

In her book, *Mama Might Be Better Off Dead*, Laurie Abraham describes the experiences of members of Jackie Banes' family with Chicago's health care system. While you will be reading the entire book, this assignment will require your in-depth consideration of only one of the people depicted in the book:

1. Robert Banes, Jackie's husband, who suffers from renal disease;

2. Cora Jackson, Jackie's grandmother, who suffers from hypertension, diabetes, and depression;

3. Tommy Markham, Jackie's father, who has hypertension; or

4. Briana, Jackie's daughter, who during the course of the book is exposed to but does not develop measles.

Please select one of these individuals as the focus of a 10-page double-spaced essay in which you address the following questions:

1. Present some background information about this individual's health problem/condition. (If this character has more than one health problem, select one health problem on which to focus your essay.) You do not need to be exhaustive in your search for information but you should be able to report (in a page) on much of the following: How widespread is this problem in the U.S. (incidence, prevalence, numbers of people affected)? Who has this problem? Who doesn't? What are the characteristics of people who seem to be at greatest risk?

2. Use the evidence presented by Abraham to identify the major socioeconomic, demographic, psychological, social, or cultural factors which seem to be influencing the health of the member of Jackie's family about whom you are writing. What one or two factors seem to have the greatest influence on this individual's health?

3. Using Andersen's model of the determinants of health service use, identify the major individual-level (predisposing, enabling, and need) factors which seem to influence this individual's use of key health services for his/her health problem.

4. Identify the major environmental or contextual factors which seem to influence this individual's use of health services. Consider both Chicago's health system as described by Abraham (including policies, institutions, and health professionals) as well as other aspects of this individual's community context which may affect his/her use of needed services.

5. You have now given full consideration to this individual's health problem and use of health services. As you know, both Medicare and many state Medicaid programs are enrolling eligibles in HMOs. Use your understanding of this member of Jackie's family, along with theory and empirical evidence considered during the semester (including papers by Perloff, Sisk et al., Ware et al., etc.), to present an assessment of how enrollment in a full-risk Health Maintenance Organization (HMO) might benefit (and/or be to the detriment) of this individual and his or her health problem. Your assessment should be balanced (considering both the positives and the negatives) and thorough, and you should draw on both social science theory and empirical evidence about HMO performance to support your assessment.

University of Vermont
Department of Social Work
Burlington, VT

Course Title: Social Work in Health (SWSS 301)
                       Fall 1998

Course Instructor: Kathleen Kirk Bishop

COURSE DESCRIPTION

Social Work in Health is the first of two required advanced-level practice courses for students who have chosen the Health/Mental Health concentration. It is intended to develop family-centered, advanced social work practitioners who can apply a variety of theoretical and empirically grounded approaches with clients and client systems in health and health-related settings. Considerable emphasis is placed on the use of students' field-based client and client system experiences in critically analyzing and evaluating the selected theoretical and empirically grounded practice paradigms for planned actions.

Within the current atmosphere of major health care restructuring and reform, the course assists students to define their discrete as well as overlapping roles in the planning, delivery, administration, and evaluation of social work services within health service delivery systems, and to use knowledge of policy, human behavior, and research to work for social justice for clients and client systems.

The course also addresses and critically analyzes some of the unique ethical dilemmas and complex practice issues which confront social workers in health settings, such as: advanced directives, genetics, HIV/AIDS, and organ transplantation.

Prerequisites: completion of foundation year curriculum, concurrent advanced year field practicum, or permission.

OBJECTIVES

Knowledge Objectives

To be able to:

- incorporate new knowledge and understanding of the personal, social, cultural, political, and economic impact of health problems and policies into social work practice with clients in health settings;
- demonstrate a conceptualization of health issues which builds on a strengths-based and ecological approach and incorporates a family-systems and family-centered approach;
- evaluate the influence of gender, race, class, age, sexual orientation, religion, and ableness on the health systems' responses to clients' health concerns;
- identify and critically analyze ethical dilemmas and complex practice issues which characterize social work practice in health settings;
- identify and critically analyze the discrete as well as overlapping roles of social workers in health settings which model family and interprofessional collaborative practice.

Values Objectives

To be able to:

- demonstrate, in the classroom and in field agencies, the ability to honor and respect the knowledge, values, and skills of clients, students, professionals, and self, in a critical analysis and evaluation of practice;

- evaluate health programs and policies through a social justice and human rights lens and demonstrate leadership in seeking an equitable distribution of resources and services to diverse groups of clients;

- demonstrate the capacity to identify and evaluate personal and professional values in relation to choice of theories, skills, and practice paradigms—in collaborative decision making and planned action with clients and other professionals;

- demonstrate the ability to critically analyze and evaluate selected complex health issues, and suggest policy and practice actions which reflect synthesis of social work values and ethics.

Skills Objectives

To be able to:

- apply a framework for social work practice which responds to the personal, social, cultural, political, and economic inequities of distribution of services and resources to diverse groups of clients;

- apply and critically evaluate a framework for practice which is strengths based, family centered, and which demonstrates a partnership with clients in selecting assessment and intervention strategies;

- provide social work leadership in the application and evaluation of frameworks for intervention to "cutting edge" and complex health issues (e.g., HIV/AIDS, advanced directives, genetics) which require multilevel and multiple professional and consumer-directed services;

- demonstrate and evaluate the ability to practice interprofessionally and collaboratively within and across varying service delivery systems;

- engage in a process of peer supervision in the classroom to critically analyze and evaluate one's own and other students' work on self, with clients and client systems in their field agencies and work settings.

SELECTED INSTRUCTOR'S ASSUMPTIONS REGARDING THE COURSE

Throughout the semester, we will work collaboratively on identifying the assumptions underlying the various theories, assessment and intervention practices, analysis and evaluation strategies, and the language used in our classes. The following represent some of the professor's assumptions in articulating the knowledge, values, and skills objectives:

A1. "From its earliest beginnings, social work practice in health care has recognized the importance of environmental factors as contributing to both the onset and successful treatment of physical illness. A significant part of the environment is the family...in which health related attitudes and behaviors are learned and which is, most frequently, the context for healing and renewal." Whitaker, J. K., 1990.

A2. "Empirical research and clinical observation provide convincing evidence that families influence significantly the health status of individual family members...on other members and on family relationships and family functioning....The call for family interventions to assist families in health promotion and illness response roles is compelling." Ell, K. & Northen, H., 1990.

Definition

Family or family members are defined to include the diversity in our family structure today, including those related legally and biologically, foster parents, surrogates, gay and lesbian families, guardians, and other families which may/may not be built on legal marriage or biological parenting (Bishop, K. K., 1990, *Family/Professional Collaboration Project*). In practice, students are encouraged to ask the people they work with to share their definition of their *family*.

    A3. Social work in health settings, by its very nature, requires collaborative and interprofessional skills.

EVALUATION OF COURSE OUTCOMES

1. Participation (see discussion under "Major Course Requirements"), which includes active participation in the classroom and in your local community whenever possible.

2. There are 3 required, written assignments which are detailed in individual assignment instruction sheets at the end of the syllabus. Each of these assignments is designed to assist you in demonstrating your mastery and integration of the knowledge, skills, and values course objectives.

3. There is 1 assignment which requires students to work in small groups to fulfill specifically the objectives related to the critical analysis, synthesis, and evaluation of a selected complex health issue—and to present this issue within the context of a staff development workshop to a group of practitioners, social workers, and others. A group-designed outline is one expected outcome.

4. Students are, as part of their participation, required to present ongoing work with clients and client systems. I am discussing this expectation separately because approximately 1/3 of class time will be spent in professor/peer supervision groups, working on self and analyzing and evaluating one's own and others' practice.

5. Students will participate in a minimum of 2 course evaluations, one at midterm and one near the end of the course. In addition, I will encourage and solicit evaluative information throughout the semester.

Additional Requirements

1. Attendance: students are expected to attend and participate in all classes. In the spirit of a practice class, I expect you to model the kinds of behavior you are using in agencies (e.g., if an emergency occurs and you must miss class, please notify me immediately and plan how you will make up the missed work). If you have a question regarding cancellation of class due to weather, I will leave that message with the Department secretaries.

2. Assignments and timeliness: students are expected to complete all written, reading, presentation, and other assignments by the deadlines in the syllabus. Any situations that could require exceptions must be discussed early. No exceptions will be made if the assignment is not handed in on time, and there has been no request for an extension. The grade for a missed assignment is an F.

3. Incompletes: it is the policy of the Graduate College to offer the final grade of incomplete only in *highly exceptional* cases. It may not be used as an extension. When an incomplete is granted, it must be completed within the negotiated time frame. The student is responsible for assuring that the paperwork is completed.

4. It is the policy of the Department of Social Work that *students may not continue in the field* with an outstanding grade of incomplete in the preceding concurrent practice course.

METHODS

Instruction and Learning Approach

    "Through dialogue, the teacher-of-the-students and the students-of-the-teacher cease to exist and a new term emerges: teacher-student and student-teacher. The teacher is no longer merely the one-who-teaches, but one who is (herself) himself taught in dialogue with students, who in turn, while being taught, also teach. They become jointly responsible for a process in which all grow...." (P. Freire, 1994). I believe that this philosophical expression of the teaching/learning methodology is appropriate for a group of advanced-level students who will be emphasizing application, critical analysis, synthesis, and evaluation in their independent and collaborative work in this course and in their field agencies.

This course will use a mix of cognitive, affective, and experiential methodology to achieve the objectives and demonstrate student outcomes. *Cognitive methods* include brief lectures (instructor, guests, students) and discussions. *Affective methods* include journaling around use of self and consultation on practice issues, student small group presentations of health issues and client material (under agreed-upon confidentiality rules) and value base analysis. *Experiential methods* include role play, student-generated exercises and presentations, family/consumer narrations, peer supervision, and field practicum.

RELATIONSHIP OF THIS COURSE TO THE REST OF THE CURRICULUM

As the first advanced practice course in the Health/Mental Health concentration, this course is taken concurrently with the first semester of the Advanced Field Practicum and builds upon the student's liberal arts perspective and the foundation knowledge, values, and skills in practice, field practicum, research, policy, and human behavior in the social environment. At the advanced level, this course emphasizes application, critical analysis, synthesis, and evaluation, and integrates learning across the advanced curriculum in policy, research, human behavior in the social environment, and students' field agency practice.

READINGS

Readings

Bishop, K. K., Woll, J., & Arango, P. (1993). *Family/professional collaboration for children with special health needs and their families.* Burlington, VT: Department of Social Work, University of Vermont. To be distributed.

Hartman, A. (Ed.). (March 1995). Social work: Challenges and directions. *Families in Society*, 75th anniversary special issue on valuing the family. Available at university bookstore.

Maternal and Child Health Bureau. (1997). *Achieving the Goals 2000: National agenda for children with special health care needs.* Rockville, MD: Author. To be distributed.

Papero, D. V. (1990). *Bowen family systems theory.* Boston: Allyn and Bacon. Available at university bookstore.

Coursepack of readings (available at university bookstore).

Recommended Readings

Bishop, K. K., Taylor, M. S., & Arango, P. (Eds.). (1997). *Partnerships at work: Lessons learned from programs and practices of families, professionals, and communities.* Burlington, VT: Department of Social Work, University of Vermont. To be distributed.

Carter, B., & McGoldrick, M. (1988). *The changing family life cycle.* New York: Garner.

Copeland, V. C. (1996). Immunization among African American children: Implications for social workers. *Health and Social Work, 21*(2), 105-114.

Davidson, K. W., & Clarke, S. S. (Eds.). (1990). *Social work in health care: A handbook for practice* (Parts I, II). Binghamton, NY: Haworth.

Dhooper, S. S. (1997). *Social work in health care in the 21st century.* Thousand Oaks, CA: Sage.

Ell, K., & Northen, H. (1990). *Families and health care: Psychosocial practice.* New York: Aldine de Gruyter.

Featherstone, H. (1980). *A difference in the family: Life with a disabled child.* New York: Basic Books.

Families in Society. (June 1992). Special issue on multicultural practice (all articles).

Germain, C. B. (1984). *Social work practice in health care: An ecological perspective.* New York: Free Press.

Gross, R., Rabinowitz, J., Feldman, D., & Boerma, W. (1996). Primary health care physician's treatment of psychosocial problems: Implications for social work. *Health and Social Work, 21*(2), 89-95.

Harper, K. V., & Lantz, J. (1996). *Cross-cultural practice: Social work with diverse populations.* Chicago: Lyceum.

Hartman, A., & Laird, J. (1983). *Family-centered social work practice.* New York: Free Press.

Health and Social Work. (August 1996). Special issue on managed care (all articles).

Hostler, S. L. (1994). *Family centered care: An approach to implementation.* Charlottesville, VA: University of Virginia, Children's Medical Center, Kluge Children's Rehabilitation Center.

Jeppson, E. S., & Thomas, J. (1993). *Essential allies: Families as advisors.* Bethesda, MD: Institute for Family-Centered Care.

Julia, M. C. (1996). *Multicultural awareness in the health care professions.* Boston: Allyn and Bacon.

Kadushin, G. (1996). Gay men with AIDS and their families of origin: An analysis of social support. *Health and Social Work, 21*(2), 141-149.

Kavanagh, K. H., & Kennedy, P. H. (1992). *Promoting cultural diversity: Strategies for health care professionals.* Thousand Oaks, CA: Sage.

Kerson, T. S., & Associates (1989). *Social work in health settings: Practice in context.* New York: Haworth.

Maternal and Child Health Bureau. (1997). *Healthy people 2000: National agenda for children with special health care needs.* Rockville, MD: Author. To be distributed.

McGoldrick, M., Pearce, J. K., & Giordano, J. (1996). *Ethnicity and family therapy.* New York: Guilford.

Miller, R. S., & Rehr, H. (1983). *Social work issues in health care.* Englewood Cliffs, NJ: Prentice Hall.

Morrow-Howell, N., Chadiha, L. A., Proctor, E. K., Hourd-Bryant, M., & Dore, P. (1996). Racial differences in discharge planning. *Health and Social Work, 21*(2), 131-139.

Peterson, M. R. (1992). *At personal risk.* New York: Norton.

Rosenberg, G., & Rehr, H. (1983). *Advancing social work practice in the health care field.* Binghamton, NY: Haworth.

Saleebey, D. (1997). *The strengths perspective in social work practice.* New York: Longman.

Shelton, T. L., & Stepanek, J. S. (1994). *Family-centered care for children with special health care needs.* Available from the Association for the Care of Children's Health, Bethesda, MD.

Sieppert, J. D. (1996). Attitudes toward and knowledge of chronic pain: A survey of medical social workers. *Health and Social Work, 21*(2), 122-130.

Singer, G. H. S., Powers, L. E., & Olson, A. L. *Redefining family support: Innovations in public-private partnerships.* Baltimore, MD: Paul H. Brookes.

Surgeon General's Report. (1987). *Children with special health care needs.* Washington, DC: U.S. Department of Health and Human Services.

Walters, M., Carter, C., Papp, P., & Silverstein, O. (1988). *The invisible web: Gender patterns in family relationships.* New York: Guilford.

Webb, N. B. (1993). *Helping bereaved children: A handbook for practitioners.* New York: Guilford.

Weiss, J. O., & Mackta, J. S. (1996). *Starting and sustaining genetic support groups.* Baltimore: Johns Hopkins University Press.

Wesley, C. A. (1996). Social work and end-of-life decisions: Self-determination and the common good. *Health and Social Work, 21*(2), 115-120.

Recommended References and Social Work Journals

> American Journal of Public Health
> Encyclopedia of Social Work
> Families in Society
> Family Voices *(a national grassroots network of families and friends speaking on behalf of children with special health care needs).*
> Harvard Women's Health Watch
> Health and Social Work
> Health and Social Policy
> Internet - various health web sites
> Journal of Family Issues
> Journal of Rural Health
> Research on Social Work Practice
> Social Work in Health Care
> The Atlantic
> (in addition to the other social work journals you have been reading)

MAJOR COURSE REQUIREMENTS AND ASSIGNMENTS

1. Active participation in all classes. Each student must be prepared to discuss readings for each class and to make presentations as required. In addition, each student will present work with clients from their field placement which illustrate complex practice issues and involve health. Students may also present work on self, using the genogram and ecomap assignment.

2. Each student's developing practice paradigm (See attached guide for assignment #2).

3. Family systems assignment: genogram, ecological assessment, intergenerational assessment which includes a history and analysis of health issues; you may choose a time period of crisis or change in your family system. See attached guide for assignment #3.

4. Group presentation and outline with references. See attached guide for assignment #4.

GRADING

The standard University of Vermont grading system for graduate courses will be used.

1. Participation (dialogue, client issues, peer supervision)   25%
2. Practice paradigm paper   30%
   (Weeks 3, 8, 14)
3. Family systems assignment   20%
   (Week 11)
4. Group presentation and written outline with references   25%
   (Weeks 11–14)

COURSE OUTLINE AND SCHEDULE

(* denotes article in purchased journal)

Unit I. Health, health delivery system, context for practice.

Week 1
Introduction to the course and to social work practice in health, exploration of the concept of health.
Required

Bartlett, H. M. (1961, revised 1988). Analysis of social work practice in any particular field. In H. M. Bartlett, *Analyzing social work practice by fields* (pp. 7-39). Silver Spring, MD: National Association of Social Workers.

Dhooper (1997), Chapter 1, Introduction, 1-48.

* Pinderhughes, E. (1995). Empowering diverse populations: Family practice in the 21st century. *Families in Society, 76,* 131-139.

Recommended

Goicoechea-Balbona, A. M. (1997). Culturally specific health care model for ensuring health care use by rural ethnically diverse families affected by HIV/AIDS. *Health and Social Work, 22,* 172-180.

Week 2
Historical context, health delivery system (structure, organization, population).
Required

Dhooper (1997), Chapter 2, Health care settings: Their past, pp. 49-94.

Germain (1984). Chapter 1. The health care system as context for social work practice. *Social work practice in health care.*

Iatridis, D. S. (1990). Cuba's health care policy: Prevention and active community participation. *Social Work, 35*(1), 29-35.

Recommended

Rehr, H. (1985, Fall). Medical care organization and the social service connection. *Health and Social Work, 10,* 245-257.

Saywell, R. M., Jr., Zollinger, T. W., Schaefer, M. E., Schmitt, T. M., & Ladd, J. K. (1993). Children with special health care needs program: Urban/rural comparisons. *The Journal of Rural Health, 9,* 314-323.

Week 3
The social work practitioner in health.
Required

Davidson, J. R., & Davidson, T. (1996). Confidentiality and managed care: Ethical and legal concerns. *Health and Social Work, 21,* 208-215.

Dhooper (1997), Chapter 3, Future Needs of Health Care, 95-130.

Ell & Northen (1990), "Social work intervention with families in health care," 121-141. New York: Aldine de Gruyter.

Recommended

Bogo, M., & colleagues. (1992). Advancing social work practice in the health field: A collaborative research partnership. *Health and Social Work, 19,* 223-235.

Rosenberg, G. (1982), "Practice roles and functions of the health social worker," in Miller & Rehr, 121-180.

Week 4

Health care reform and financing: Where are we going?

Required

Students will use the Internet to find, read, and comment on the most current information on health care reform and financing. They will also examine their personal health care financing system.

Callahan, J. (1996). Documentation of client dangerousness in a managed care environment. *Health and Social Work*, 21, 202-207.

Gorin, S. (1997). Universal health care coverage in the United States: Barriers, prospects, and implications. *Health and Social Work*, 22, 223-230.

Recommended

Keigher, S. M. (1994). The morning after deficit reduction: The poverty of U.S. maternal and child health policy. *Health and Social Work*, *19*, 143-147.

Lundblad, K. S. (1995). Jane Addams and social reform: A role model for the 1990s. *Social Work*, *40*, 661-669.

Perloff, J. D. (1996). Medicaid managed care and urban poor people: Implications for social work. *Health and Social Work*, *21*, 189-194.

Poole, D. L. (1996). Editorial: Keeping managed care in balance. *Health and Social Work*, *21*, 163-165.

Unit II.   Health and families, family-centered practice, health from a family systems perspective.

Week 5

Families talk with social work students about health and family-centered practice.
Guest Lecturers: Family Members; Parent to Parent of Vermont (materials to be distributed)

Required

Bishop, Woll, & Arango (1993).

* Hartman, A. (1995). Ideological themes in family policy. *Families in Society*, *76*, 182-192.

* Weick, A., & Saleebey, D. (1995). Supporting family strengths: Orienting policy and practice toward the 21st century. *Families in Society*, *76*, 141-149.

Recommended

Cole, E. S. (1995). Becoming family-centered: Child welfare's challenge. *Families in Society*, *76*, 163-172.

Featherstone (1980).

Hall, S. R. (1996). The community-centered model of managed care for people with developmental disabilities. *Health and Social Work*, 21, 225-229.

Week 6

The genetic connection: What social workers need to know.

Required

Bishop, K. K. (1993). Psychosocial aspects of genetic disorders: Implications for practice. *Families in Society*, *74*, 207-212.

Weiss, J. O. (1993). Genetic disorders: Support groups and advocacy. *Families in Society*, *74*, 213-220.

Wertz, D. C., Fanos, J. H., & Reilly, P. R. (1994). Genetic testing for children and adolescents: Who decides? *Journal of the American Medical Association*, *272*, 875-880.

Recommended

Bernhardt, B., & Rauch, J. B. (1993). Genetic family histories: An aid to social work assessment. *Families in Society*, *74*, 195-206.

Elmer-DeWitt, P. (1994, Jan. 17). Genetics: The future is now. *Time*, pp. 47-53.

Murray, T. H. (1992). Genetics and the moral mission of health insurance. *Hastings Center Report*, 12-16. New York: Hastings Center.

Nash, J. M. (1994, Jan. 17). Riding the DNA trail. *Time*, pp. 54-55.

Week 7
Family-centered and family systems theory for practice.

Required

Anderson, S. C. (1995). Education for family-centered practice. *Families in Society*, *76*, 163-181.

Hartman, A. (1995). Diagrammatic assessment of family relationships. *Families in Society*, *76*, 111-122.

McGoldrick, M., & Gerson, R. (1985). Why genograms? In M. McGoldrick & R. Gerson, *Genograms in family assessment*, 1-8. New York: Norton.

Recommended

Van Hook, M. P., Berkman, B., & Dunkle, R. (1996). Assessment tools for general health care settings: PRIME-MD, OARS, and SF-36. *Health and Social Work*, 21, 230-234.

Review of genogram, culturagram and ecomap tools, outlines to guide data-gathering, and genogram interpretive categories (handouts) and class exercises with tools.

Week 8

Required

Laird, J. (1995). Family-centered practice in the postmodern era. *Families in Society*, *76*, 150-162.

Papero, D. V. (1990). *Bowen family systems theory*. Boston: Allyn and Bacon.

Chapter 1: Bowen theory in perspective, 1-19

Chapter 2: The family as a unit, 21-35

Chapter 3: Bowen family systems theory, 37-64

Week 9

Required

Papero, D. V. (1990). *Bowen family systems theory*. Boston: Allyn and Bacon.

Chapter 4: Family systems theory in clinical practice, 67-81

Chapter 5: The clinical situation: The "B" family, 83-97

Chapter 6: Training in theory, thought, and therapy, 99-109

Wynne, L. C., Shields, C. G., & Sirkin, M. I. (1992). Illness, family theory, and family therapy: Conceptual issues. *Family Process*, 31, 3-18.

Unit III. Health and social work practice issues, functions, and roles.

Weeks 10, 11, 12, 13, 14
Topics and reading assignments for this unit are student-generated in collaboration with the professor. As soon as groups are formed and topics and readings have been chosen, they will be added to our syllabus.

See assignment #4 for examples of students' work from Fall 1995 and 1996

Unit IV. Social work and health in the 21st century.

Week 15
Health Issues in the 21st Century
Interprofessional Collaborative Practice
Readings to be assigned
Course Evaluation

APPENDIX

ASSIGNMENT #2—DEVELOPING PRACTICE PARADIGM

As second-year students in the concentration year of the graduate social work program, it is important to continue to define, describe, and be able to explain what constitutes your developing practice paradigm. That is, what are the philosophical beliefs and values that guide your practice with people and systems? How would you describe the elements of your practice?

How do you think about the issues that your clients and service systems present? What guides your thinking? How do you think about what to do? How do you do it? What guides how you approach and work with clients and client systems? These are questions to help you think about your practice. They are not the only questions you might want to ask yourself and they are not necessarily the "right" questions to ask.

Draft #1 due Week 3
Draft #2 due Week 8
Final draft paradigm paper due on or before Week 14.

ASSIGNMENT #3—FAMILY SYSTEMS ASSIGNMENT

In fulfillment of course objectives related to: the ecological perspective, health as a family systems issue, developing an understanding of/application of a family-centered and culturally appropriate perspective—and including the important issue of developing a continuing awareness of self within the client situation, students will develop the following:

- a minimum of a three-generation genogram, using the McGoldrick schema for drawing genograms (handout);
- an ecomap, using the Hartman and Laird approach (Family-Centered Social Work Practice, Chapter 8, The Family in Space: Ecological Assessment).

For this assignment, students may choose a time period of crisis or change in your family system which includes a history and analysis of health issues. In approximately 5 pages, use selected concepts from Bowen Family Systems theory to interpret your family genogram and ecomap. Include family, cultural, and ethnic issues, and demonstrate a connection to family-centered principles. Suggest strategies and family maneuvers that you might make in attempting to differentiate self within your family system, etc. Be daring, creative, responsible, and analytical!

Assignment due Week 11

(Although I believe that you will learn the most about self and make more progress on your personal issues by using your family of origin, no student is required to use their own family. Please see me regarding an alternate way to complete this assignment if you choose not to use your family of origin.)

ASSIGNMENT #4—SOCIAL WORK ISSUES PRESENTATION

Students, using a small work group format (not to exceed 4 students per group), will select an issue and plan a presentation that would be appropriate in an agency setting. Some suggested issues are:

interprofessional collaboration	lead poisoning
managed care	rape services in health care organizations
*HIV/AIDS	rural adolescent health services
*advanced directives	home health services for the elderly
organ transplant clinics	assisted suicide

(* strongly recommended for selection)

You must develop the context for this presentation (e.g., who is the audience, what is the setting), a set of outcome objectives, a minimum of 3 required readings, and a written evaluation form for your presentation. Please administer this evaluation to the class immediately following your presentation and provide a copy of the evaluations to the Professor when you hand in your outline and readings.

The time period for the presentations *may not exceed 75 minutes.*

Creativity and mixed media should be considered for the presentation, e.g., overheads, slides, films, lecture, guest lecturers, exercises, case examples, etc.

Each student group should plan a short meeting with the Professor which will include a written plan and co-selected readings to be assigned for the presentation. (This meeting should occur a minimum of three weeks before the presentation is scheduled.)

Examples of Group Presentation Topics and Readings (Fall 1995 and 1996)

Advanced Directives

Guest Presenter: Arnold Golodetz, M.D.

Freedman, M. (1994). Helping home bound elderly clients understand and use advanced directives. *Social Work in Health Care,* 20, 61-73.

Lerer, G. (1994). Social work's role in a case of withdrawal of basic life supports. *Social Work in Health Care,* 20, 109-115.

Vermont Ethics Network. (1995). *Taking steps: To plan for critical health care decisions* (brochure). Montpelier, VT: Author.

As part of your assignment for today please complete the values section of *Taking Steps.* In addition, please bring all assigned reading to class, especially the *Taking Steps* brochure. We will begin our advanced directives documents in class.

HIV/AIDS

Geballe, S., Gruenael, J., & Andiman, W. (Eds.). (1995). *Forgotten children of the AIDS epidemic.* New Haven, CT: Yale University Press.

Gillman, R. (1991). From resistance to rewards: Social workers' experiences and attitudes toward AIDS. *Families in Society,* 12, 593-601.

Gostin, K. (1991). The needle-borne HIV epidemic: Causes and public health responses. *Behavioral Sciences and the Law,* 9, 287-304.

Nagler, S. F., Adnopoz, J., & Forsyth, B. W. (1995). Uncertainty, stigma, and secrecy: Psychological aspects of AIDS for children and adolescents. In S. Geballe, et al. (Eds.), *Forgotten children of the AIDS epidemic.* New Haven, CT: Yale University Press.

Rounds, K. A. (1988). AIDS in rural areas: Challenges to providing care. *Social Work,* May/June, 257-261.

The issue of competence/incompetence when working with elders who are cognitively impaired.
Guest Presenter: Jane Rheaume, MSW, Social Worker—Addison County Home Health

Rathbone-McCuan, E. (1992). Aged adult protective services clients: People of unrecognized potential. In D. Saleebey (Ed.), *The strengths perspective in social work practice* (pp. 98-110). White Plains, NY: Longman.

Longres, J. F. (1994). Self-neglect and social control: A modest test of an issue. *Journal of Gerontological Social Work, 22*(3/4), 3-20.

Kelly, T. B. (1994). Paternalism and the marginally competent: An ethical dilemma, no easy answers. *Journal of Gerontological Social Work, 23,* 67-84.

Poulin, J. E., Walker, J. L., & Walter, C. A. (1994). Interdisciplinary team membership: A survey of gerontological social workers. *Journal of Gerontological Social Work, 22,* 93-106.

COMMON COLLEGE GOALS

This course will address the following common goals adopted by The College of Education and Social Services during the Spring of 1988.

1. The Instructor and Participants will use professional concepts, theoretical terms, and scholarly understandings in communication with each other.

2. The Instructor and Participants will use problem-solving approaches to address professional problems in the study of their own practice.

3. The Instructor and Participants will advance the cause of democratic values.

4. The Instructor and Participants will deal reflectively with the enduring issues and the complex questions of the day.

5. The Instructor and Participants will advocate for the interests of children and families.

6. The Instructor and Participants will participate fully in the obligations of their professional roles.

7. The Instructor and Participants will collaborate with colleagues in working toward common goals.

NASW CODE OF ETHICS: SUMMARY OF MAJOR PRINCIPLES

1. To maintain high standards of personal conduct and professional integrity.

2. To show primary responsibility to the client while fostering self-determination and respecting the privacy of the client.

3. To treat colleagues and their clients with respect, courtesy, fairness and professional consideration.

4. To adhere to the commitments made to the employing organizations.

5. To uphold and advance the values, ethics and knowledge of the profession.

6. To promote the general welfare of society.

Columbia University
School of Social Work
New York, NY

Course Title: Health Care Issues, Policies, and Programs (T6910:01-03)
             Fall 1998

Course Instructors: Barbara J. Berkman (chair), Teresa Gardian, Margherita DiCenzo Jellinek,
             Ji Seon Lee, & Darrell Wheeler

DESCRIPTION

The overall goal of this course is to provide students with knowledge about the policies, programs, and service delivery system relevant to the health practice field and to its client systems. The course also aims to help students understand the ever-changing organizational structure of today's health care field and strengthen the students' ability to understand their role(s) as social workers in health care settings.

Attention will be given to the social policies that authorize, support, and sanction U.S. health services and the institutional delivery system(s) that host and provide these services. Throughout the course, an emphasis will be placed on understanding differential patterns of health care utilization and delivery based on demographic characteristics and on evaluating issues of accessibility, acceptability, accountability, research, ethics, and multidisciplinary care.

OBJECTIVES

To enable the student:

- To recognize the relationship between social policy and health organizational structures—federal, state, and local—as they effect the planning and implementation of health and social work services.

- To recognize the social, economic, and personal factors affecting well-being, illness, disabilities, and mental retardation of individuals and families.

- To identify factors such as ethnicity, race, gender, sociocultural variables, economics, and geographic characteristics that may affect health service delivery and/or utilization, and to apply this knowledge to developing policies and programs to meet individual and family needs.

- To develop familiarity with a range of interventive social work strategies congruent with contemporary fiscal, legal, and organizational sanctions and constraints in various health care settings.

- To identify and assess viable policy entry points for the improvement of health care to consumers attempting to negotiate a complex fragmented health care system.

- To develop the critical capacity to help in the formulation and innovation of and/or advocacy for appropriate change.

- To become familiar with methodological approaches and research designs that assess and evaluate the impact of policy on social work service delivery in the health field.

- To examine the impact of policy on organizational structures of social services and social work departments within hierarchical health delivery systems.

STATEMENT OF ADHERENCE TO UNIVERSITY AND SCHOOL POLICIES

The instructors adhere to university and school policies regarding accommodations for students with disabilities, religious holidays, incompletes, plagiarism, and students' evaluation of the course and its instruction as stated in the CUSSW Student Handbook and the CUSSW Bulletin.

TEXTS

Required

* Class Reader—T6910, Fall 1998.

* Class website: https://www1.columbia.edu/sec/itc/ssw/t6910-001/ (review on a regular basis) *[Editor's note: this site is password protected.]*

Recommended

* Blank, R.H. (1997). Price of Life: The Future of American Health Care. New York: Columbia University Press.

* Bracht, N.F. (Ed.). (1978). Social Work in Health Care: A Guide to Professional Practice. Binghamton, NY: Haworth.

* Dhooper, S.S. (1997). Social Work in Health Care in the 21st Century. Thousand Oaks, CA: Sage.

* Dumont, M.P. (1992). Treating the Poor. Belmont, MA: Dymphna Press.

* Longest, B.B., Jr. (1994). Health Policymaking in the United States. Ann Arbor, MI: AUPHA Press.

* Mechanic, D. (1989). Mental Health and Social Policy (3rd ed.). Englewood Cliffs, NJ: Prentice Hall.

* Payer, L. (1988). Medicine and Culture. New York: Penguin.

* Sparer, M.S. (1996). Medicaid and the Limits of State Health Reform. Philadelphia: Temple University Press.

* Starr, P. (1982). The Social Transformation of American Medicine. New York: Basic Books.

REQUIREMENTS

* Assignment #1—40% of grade—due Session 7
* Assignment #2—30% of grade—due Session 15
* Assignment #3—20% of grade—due Session 15

Other

Regular class attendance, peer participation, and work completion is expected—10% of grade (extenuating circumstances should be discussed with your workshop instructor).

ASSIGNMENTS

Assignment #1—Written Assignment—Due Session 7

In this assignment you are to describe your field placement with a focus on its role as a service delivery setting. This assignment is to be typed, double-spaced. The body of the text should not exceed eight pages, including references. References in the body of the paper and the reference list are to be cited using the American Psychological Association (APA) 4th edition guidelines.

Content areas to be included in this assignment include:

* Who authorizes your department or agency to perform its functions (legitimizing bodies)?

* What source(s) fund your department or agency?

* Who staffs the department or agency?

* What is the role of social work in your department or agency?

* What is the formal administrative structure of your department or agency?

* What is your department or agency's role in the health/mental health delivery system (select local community or NYC metropolitan area)?

* What major legislative changes occurred within the last five years have effected your department or agency service provision and social work role?

For students placed in multipurpose settings, discuss your working unit (department rather than hospital, clinic rather than hospital, etc.). References to the larger setting may also be included, but ensure that your written assignment distinguishes between the two as you shift between them.

Assignment #2—Website Resulting From Student Group Work—Due Session 15

For this assignment, students work in groups and select a federally legislated U.S. policy. The policy should have legislative activity within the last three years, and should have direct impact on the provision, planning, and/or evaluation of health services in the United States. All topics are to be approved by the instructor for appropriateness.

The website should include the following information:

* Identify the legislation, its name and public law number, year of enactment, year of implementation

* Identify significant historical elements associated with this act's implementation (i.e., provide a brief overview of significant social, political, and economic conditions at work as this Act is being developed)

* Briefly identify the key factors addressed by this act (i.e., who or what services are targeted; ratification of prior acts; major shifts in ideologies or practices)

* Summarize factors which facilitated the implementation of this act

* Briefly, identify unintended consequences of the legislation

* Summarize the evaluation component for this act; where there is no evaluation component, summarize the impact of this omission.

Assignment #3 Written Memorandum—Due Session 15

This written memorandum is to be prepared by each student as his/her individual assessment of the legislative act to be presented in Assignment #2. In this assignment, students should include the following information:

* Background of act (one paragraph)

* Social work services and population(s) impacted by the act (limit to three paragraphs) and an assessment of positives and negatives of each impact (limit to one or two paragraphs)

* Recommendations of possible changes needed in the Act in order to address the negatives

* This assignment is to be typed, single-spaced, and not to exceed two pages in length. Provide a reference list. Hand in at the time of the website presentation and be prepared to discuss your conclusions at that time.

SCHEDULE

Session 1
* Introduction to course, *Professor Berkman*
* Introduction to health care policy, *Professor Lee*

Session 2
* Workshops—Policy, formulation, *Professors Gardian, Jellinek, Lee*

Session 3
* Health care policy: Overview of key issues and their impact on social work practice, *Professor Lee*

Session 4
* Workshops—Health care policy, *Professors Gardian, Jellinek, Lee*

Session 5
* Diversity and minority health policy issues, *Professor Gardian*
* Mental health policy and social work health care practice, *Professor Gardian*

Session 6
* Workshops—Health care needs of diverse and minority populations, as related to mental health policy issues, *Professors Gardian, Jellinek, Lee*

Session 7
* Federal Depository: Information superhighway, *Professor Lee and Jerry Breeze (Federal Depository librarian)*

Session 8
* Workshops—Begin developing the group website assignments relating to health acts and their implications for Social Work practice, *Professors Gardian, Jellinek, Lee*

Session 9
* Election Day—no class

Session 10
* Health care needs of special populations, *Professor Wheeler*
* Ethics and values in health and mental health, *Professor Jellinek (Workshop activity will be included in this lecture)*

Session 11
* Health policy as related to developmental issues, *Professor Jellinek*

Session 12
* Workshops—The impact of health and mental health policy on developmental issues, *Professors Gardian, Jellinek, Lee*

Session 13
* Public health policy issues for social work practice in health care, *Professor Wheeler*
* Strategies for social work evaluation and research on impact of health policy, *Professor Berkman*

Session 14
* Workshops—Public Health and research policy, *Professors Gardian, Jellinek, Wheeler*

Session 15
* Website presentations, wrap-up, and celebration

SUGGESTED READINGS
Grouped by Area of Focus
(Note: RP signifies Reading Packet)

Readings with Significant Materials in a Variety of Areas

*   Aaron, H.J. Serious and Unstable Condition: Financing America's Health Care. Washington, DC: Brookings Institution, 1991.

*   Abraham, L.K. Mama Might be Better Off Dead: The Failure of Health Care in America. Chicago: University of Chicago Press, 1993.

*   Bayer, R. Private Acts, Social Consequences: AIDS and the Politics of Public Health. New York: Free Press, 1989.

*   Brown, S.S. (ed.). Prenatal Care: Reaching Mother, Reaching Infants. Washington, DC: National Academy Press, 1988.

*   Butler, P., Too Poor to be Sick. Washington, DC: American Public Health Association, 1988.

*   Callahan, D. Setting Limits: Medical Goals in an Aging Society. New York: Touchstone, 1987.

*   Dumont, M.P. Treating the Poor. Belmont, MA: Dymphna Press, 1992.

*   Fogel, B.S. et al. (eds.) Mental Health Policy for Older Americans: Protecting Minds at Risk. Washington, DC: American Psychiatric Press, 1990.

*   Freeman, H., and Levine, S. (eds.) Handbook of Medical Sociology, 4th ed. Englewood Cliffs, NJ: Prentice Hall, 1989.

*   Ginzberg, E. The Road to Reform: The Future of Health Care in America. New York: Free Press, 1994.

*   Gitterman, A., Black, R., and Stein, F. (eds.) Public Health Social Work in Maternal and Child Health Care: A Forward Plan. Proceedings: June 23-26, 1985, Division of Maternal and Child Health, Bureau of Health Care Delivery and Assistance, Health Resources Administration, U.S. Public Health Services.

*   Gostin, L.O. (ed.). AIDS and the Health Care System. New Haven: Yale University Press, 1990.

*   Loewenberg, F.M., and Dolgoff, R. Ethical Decisions for Social Work Practice, 4th ed. Itasca, IL: F.E. Peacock, 1992.

*   Mechanic, D. Mental Health and Social Policy, 3rd ed. Englewood Cliffs, NJ: Prentice Hall, 1989.

*   Payer, L. Medicine and Culture. New York: Penguin Books, 1988.

*   Rosenberg, G., and Weissman, A. (eds.) Social Work in Ambulatory Care. New York: Hawthorne Press, 1994.

*   Shapiro, J.P. No Pity: People with Disabilities Forging a New Civil Rights Movement. New York: Times Books, 1993.

*   Sparer, M.S. Medicaid and the Limits of State Health Reform. Philadelphia: Temple University Press, 1996.

*   Starr, P. The Social Transformation of American Medicine. New York: Basic Books, 1982.

I. Introduction: Linking Health and Mental Health—Social Work's Place in the Health System

*   Black, R. "Looking Ahead: Social Work as a Core Health Profession," Health and Social Work, Spring 1984, 85-95.

*   Blumenfield, S., and Rosenberg, G. "Towards a Network of Social Health Services: Redefining Discharge Planning and Expanding the Social Work Domain," Social Work in Health Care, 13(4) 1988, 31-48.

*   Dolgoff, R.L. "Clinicians as Social Policymakers," Social Casework, May 1981, 62(5), 284-292.

*   Donnelly, J.P. "A Frame for Defining Social Work in a Hospital Setting," Social Work in Health Care, 1992, 18(1), 107-119.

*   Fox, R.C. "The Medicalization and Demedicalization of American Society," Daedalus, Winter 1977, 106(1), 9-22. (RP)

*   Henk, M. Social Work in Primary Care. Newbury Park, CA: Sage, 1989.

*   Rehr, H. "Medical Care Organization and the Social Service Connection," Health and Social Work, Fall 1985, 10(4), 245-257.

* Scott, R.A., Aiken, L.H., Mechanic, D.A., and Moravcsik, J. "Organizational Aspects of Caring," Milbank Quarterly, 1995, 73(1), 77-95. (RP)

* Social Work in Health Care, volume 20(1), 1994, special issue: Social Work in Ambulatory Care: New Implications for Health and Social Services.

* Wintersteen, R.T. "Rehabilitating the Chronically Mentally Ill: Social Worker's Claim to Leadership," Social Work (31:5) October 1986, 332-337.

II. Ideologies and Values — Definitions of Health and Illness

* Caras, S. "Disabled: One More Label," Hospital and Community Psychiatry, April 1994, 45(4), 323-324. (RP)

* Engel, G. "The Clinical Application of the Biopsychosocial Model," American Journal of Psychiatry, May 1980, 535-554. (RP)

* Engel, G.L. "The Need for a New Medical Model: A Challenge for Biomedicine," Science, (196:4286), April 8, 1997, 129-136.

* Kutchins, H., and Kirk, S.A. "DSM-III-R: The Conflict over New Psychiatric Diagnoses, Health and Social Work, May 1989, 14, 91-101.

* Kane, R.A. "Lessons for Social Work from the Medical Model: A Viewpoint for Practice," Social Work, July 1982, 315-321.

* Shannon, M.T. "Health Promotion and Illness Prevention: A Biopsychosocial Perspective," Health and Social Work, (14:1) February 1989, 32-40.

* Starr, P. The Social Transformation of American Medicine. Book I, Chapters 3–5, pp. 79-197.

* Weiner, H. "An Integrative Model of Health, Illness and Disease," Health and Social Work, (9:4), Fall 1984, pp. 253-259.

III. Public Health Perspectives and Techniques

* Bromberger, J.T., and Costello, E.J. "Epidemiology of Depression for Clinicians," Social Work, 1992, 37(2), 120-125.

* Hinman, A.R. "1889 to 1989: A Century of Health and Disease," Public Health Reports, July-August 1987, 102(4), 374-380.

* Rhoades, E.R., et al. "The Indian Burden of Illness and Future Health Interventions," Public Health Reports, July-August 1987, 102(4), 361-368.

* Watkins, E. "The Conceptual Base for Public Health Social Work," Public Health Social Work in Maternal and Child Health Care: A Forward Plan (Gitterman, A., Black, R., and Stein, F., eds.), Proceedings June 23-26, 1985, Division of Maternal and Child Health, Bureau of Health Care Delivery and Assistance, Health Resources Administration, U.S. Public Health Services, 17-30.

* Whitman, B.Y., and Hennelly, V.D. "The Uses of Epidemiological Methods as the Bridge Between Prevention and Social Work Practice," Social Work in Health Care, 1982, 7(4), 27-38. (RP)

* Williams, C.L., and Berry, J.W. "Primary Prevention of Acculturative Stress Among Refugees," American Psychologist, June 1991, 46(6), 632-641.

IV. Health Care Policy and Programs

Health Policy and Health Care Reform

* Aaron, H.J. Serious Unstable Condition: Financing America's Health Care. Washington, DC: The Brookings Institution, 1991.

* Butler, P.A. Too Poor to be Sick. Washington DC: American Public Health Association, 1988.

* Fein, R. Medical Care, Medical Costs: The Search for a Health Insurance Policy. Cambridge, MA: Harvard, 1989.

* Fox, D.M. "Policy and Epidemiology: Financing Health Services for the Chronically Ill and Disabled, 1930-1990," The Milbank Quarterly, 67 (Supplement 2, Part 2), 1989, 257-287.

* Ginzberg, E. The Road to Reform: The Future of Health Care in America. New York: Free Press, 1994.

* Kane, R.A. "Health Policy and Social Workers in Health: Past, Present, and Future," Health and Social Work, (10:4) Fall, 1985, 258-270.

* Kane, R.A. Expanding the Home Care Concept: Blurring Distinctions among Home Care, Institutional Care, and Other Long-Term-Care Services," Milbank Quarterly, 1995, 73(2), 161-186.

* Kane, R.A., and Kane, R.L. "What is Long-Term Care?" (ch. 1); "The Current State of Long-Term Care," (ch. 3) "Long-Term Care Issues: Quality, Assess and Cost," (ch. 4), "Synthesizing the Evidence," (ch. 11), "Improving Long-Term Care: Next Steps," (ch. 12) Long Term Care, Principles, Programs, and Policies.

* Koyanagi, C., Manes, J., Surles, R., and Goldman, H.H. "On Being Very Smart: The Mental Health Community's Response in the Health Care Reform Debate," Hospital and Community Psychiatry, June 1993, 44(6), 537-542.

* Oberg, C.H., and Polich, C.L. "Medicaid: Entering the Third Decade," Health Affairs, Fall 1988, 7(3), 83-96.

* Santiago, J.M. "The Fate of Mental Health Services in Health Reform: I. A System in Crisis and II. Realistic Solutions." Hospital and Community Psychiatry, November 1992, 43(11), 1091-1099.

* Shortell, S.M., Gillies, R.R., and Devers, K.J. "Reinventing the American Hospital," Milbank Quarterly, 1995, 73(2), 131-160. (RP)

* Stoeckle, J.D. "The Citadel Cannot Hold: Technologies Go Outside the Hospital, Patients, and Doctors Too," Milbank Quarterly, 1995, 73(1), 3-17. (RP)

* Starr, P. The Social Transformation of American Medicine, Book II, Chapters 3, 4,., and 5, pp. 335-449. New York: Basic Books.

* Webber, H.S. "The Failure of Health-Care Reform: An Essay Review," Social Service Review, June 1995, 69(4), 309-322. (RP)

V. Racial and Socioeconomic Differences in Health Access and Health Status

* Davis, K., Blanton, M.L., Lyons, B., Mullan, F., Powe, N., and Rowland, D., "Health Care for Black Americans: The Public Sector Role," Milbank Quarterly, 1987, (65: Supplement 1), 213-247.

* Feinstein, J.S. "The Relationship between Socioeconomic Status and Health: A Review of the Literature," Milbank Quarterly, 1993, 71(1), 279-322.

* Laveist, T.A. "Segregation, Poverty and Empowerment: Health Consequences for African Americans," Milbank Quarterly, 1993, 71(1), 41-64.

* Peter, R.F., Newacheck, P.W., and Halfon, N. "Access to Care for Poor Children: Separate and Unequal?" Journal of the American Medical Association, May 27, 1992, 267(20), 2760-2764. (RP)

* Wade, J.C. "Institutional Racism: An Analysis of the Mental Health System," American Journal of Orthopsychiatry, October 1993, 63(4), 536-544. (RP)

VI. Health Policy and Programs—Selected Target Populations

Maternal, Child, and Adolescent Health

* American Journal of Public Health. Special issues on "Women's Health," February and May 1992, volume 82(2, 5): "Children's and Adolescents' Health," March 1992, 82(3).

* Carlton. T.O., and Poole, D.L. "Trends in Maternal and Child Health Care: Implications for Research and Issues for Social Work Practice," Social Work in Health Care, 1990, 15(1), 45-62.

* Gehlert, S., and Lickey, S. "Social and Health Policy Concerns Raised by the Introduction of the Contraceptive Norplant," Social Service Review, June 1995, 69(4), 323- 227. (RP)

* Health and Social Work. Special issue on women and children, May 1994, 19(2).

Prenatal and Perinatal Issues

* Bassuk, E.L., and Weinreb, L. "Homeless Pregnant Women: Two Generations at Risk," American Journal of Orthopsychiatry, July 1993, 63(3), 348-357.

* Belville, R. et al. "The Community as a Strategic Site for Refining High Perinatal Risk Assessments and Interventions," Social Work in Health Care, 1991, 16(1), 5-19. (RP)

* Brown, S., Prenatal Care: Reaching Mothers: Reaching Infants. Washington DC: Institute of Medicine, National Academy Press, 1988.

* Combs-Orme, T. "Infant Mortality and Social Work: Legacy of Success," Social Service Review, March 1988, 62(1), 83-102.

* Joyce, T., "The Dramatic Increase in the Rate of Low Birthweight in New York City: An Aggregate Time-Series Analysis," American Journal of Public Health, June 1990, 80(6), 682-684.

* Kotch, J.B., Blakely, C.H., Brown, S.S., and Wong, F.Y. A Pound of Prevention: The Case for Universal Maternity Care in the U.S. Washington, DC: American Public Health Association, 1992.

* Schaffer, M.A., and Lia-Hoagberg, B. "Prenatal Care Among Low-Income Women," Families in Society, March 1994, 152-159.

* Walther, V.N. "Emerging Roles of Social Work in Perinatal Services," Social Work in Health Care, 1990, 15(2), 35-48.

* Yankauer, A. "What Infant Mortality Tells Us," American Journal of Public Health, June 1990, 80(6), 653-654. (RP)

Access to Child Health Services

* Berkowitz, G., Halfon, N., Klee, L. "Improving Access to Health Care: Case Management for Vulnerable Children," Social Work in Health Care, 1992, 17(1), 101-123.

* Peter, R.F., Newacheck, P.W., and Halfon, N. "Access to Care for Poor Children: Separate and Unequal?" Journal of the American Medical Association, May 27, 1992, 267(20), 2760-2764.

Prenatal Drug Exposure

* Gustavsson, N.S. "Drug Exposed Infants and their Mothers: Facts, Myths, and Needs," Social Work in Health Care, 1992, 16(4), 87-100.

* Scherling, D. "Prenatal Cocaine Exposure and Childhood Psychopathology: A Developmental Analysis," American Journal of Orthopsychiatry, January 1994, 64(1), 9-19.

Adolescent Health and Pregnancy

* Combs-Orme, T. "Health Effects of Adolescent Pregnancy: Implications for Social Workers," Families in Society, June 1993, 74(6), 344-354.

* Harold, R.D., and Harold, N.B. "School-Based Clinics: A Response to the Physical and Mental Health Needs of Adolescents," Health and Social Work, 1993, 18(1), 65-74.

* Plotnick, R.P. "The Effects of Social Policies on Teenage Pregnancy and Childbearing," Families in Society, June 1993, 74(6), 324-328.

Child Mental Health Issues

* LeCroy, C.W. "Enhancing the Delivery of Effective Mental Health Services to Children," Social Work, 1992, 37(3), 225-231.

* LeCroy, C.W., and Ashford, J.B. 1992. "Children's Mental Health: Current Findings and Research Directions," Social Work Research and Abstracts, 1992, 28, 13-20.

* Lourie, I.S., and Katz-Leavy, J. "New Directions for Mental Health Services for Families and Children," Families in Society, 1991, 227-285.

* Rothman, S. Woman's Proper Place: A History of Changing Ideals and Practices, 1870 to the Present. New York: Basic Books, 1978.

* Trupin, E.W., Forsyth-Stephens, A., and Low, B.P. "Service Needs of Severely Disturbed Children," American Journal of Public Health, August 1991, 81(8), 975-980.

Mothers Who Are Mentally Ill

* Apfel, R.J., and Handel, M.II. Madness and Loss of Motherhood: Sexuality, Reproduction, and Long-Term Mental Illness. Washington, DC: American Psychiatric Press, 1993.

* Coverdale, J.H., Bayer, T.L., McCullough, L.B., and Chervenak, F.A. "Respecting the Autonomy of Chronic Mentally Ill Women in Decisions About Contraception," Hospital and Community Psychiatry, July 1993, 44(7), 671-674.

* Nicholson, J., Geller, J.L., Fisher, W.H., and Dion, G.L. "State Policies and Programs that Address the Needs of Mentally Ill Mothers in the Public Sector," Hospital and Community Psychiatry, May 1993, 44(5), 484-489.

* Oyserman, D., Mowbray, C.T., and Zemencuk, J.K. "Resources and Supports for Mothers with Severe Mental Illness," Health and Social Work, May 1994, 19(2), 132-142.

Women's Health

* Olson, M.M., "Introduction: Reclaiming the 'Other'—Women, Health Care and Social Work," Social Work in Health Care, 1994, 19(3/4), 1-16.

* Millner, L., and Widerman, E. "Women's Health Issues: A Review of the Current Literature in the Social Work Journal, 1985-1992," Social Work in Health Care, 1994, 19(3/4), 145-172.

* Sexhzer, J.A., Giffin, A., and Pfafflin, S. Forging a Women's Health Research Agenda. New York: New York Academy of Sciences, 1994.

Disability Issues and Rights; Children with Chronic Illnesses and Disabilities

* Batavia, A.I. "Health Care Reform and People with Disabilities," Health Affairs, April 1993, 12(1), 40-57.

* Black, R.B., and Weiss, J.O. "Chronic Physical Illness and Disability." In A. Gitterman, ed. Handbook of Social Work Practice with Vulnerable Populations, pp. 137-164. New York: Columbia University Press, 1991.

* Gliedman, J., and Roth, W., The Unexpected Minority—Handicapped Children in America. New York: Harcourt, Brace and Jovanovich, 1980, Chapters 1-3.

* Hauser-Cram, P., Upshur, C., Krauss, M., and Shonkoff, J.P. "Implications of Public Law 99-457 for Early Intervention Services for Infants and Toddlers with Disabilities," Social Policy Report, Autumn 1988, III(3), 1-16.

* Hobbs, N., Perrin, J.M., and Ireys, H.T. Chronically Ill Children and their Families. San Fransico: Jossey-Bass, 1985.

* Jones, N.L. "Essential Requirements of the Act: A Short History and Overview." In J. West, ed. The Americans with Disabilities Act: From Policy to Practice. Milbank Quarterly, 1991, 69 (Supplements 1/2), 25-54.

* Meisels, S.J. "Meeting the mandate of Public Law 99-457: Early Childhood Intervention in the Nineties," American Journal of Orthopsychiatry, July 1989, 59(3), 451-460.

VII. AIDS

* American Journal of Public Health. Special issue on HIV/AIDS, April 1992, 82(4).

* Bayer, R. Private Acts, Social Consequences: AIDS and the Politics of Public Health. New York: Free Press, 1989 (Chapters 1 and 8).

* Brennan, J.P. "HIV/AIDS: Implications for Health Care Reform," Families in Society, June 1994, 75(6), 385-392. (RP)

† Gostin, L.O. (ed.). AIDS and the Health Care System. New Haven: Yale University Press, 1990.

* Jimenez, M.A., and Jimenez, D.R. "Latinos and HIV Disease: Issues, Practice, and Policy Implications," Social Work in Health Care, 1992, 17(2), 41-51.

* Ozawa, M.N., Auslander, W.F., and Slonim-Nevo, V. "Problems in Financing the Care of AIDS Patients," Social Work, July 1993, 38(4), 369-377.

* Roberts, C.S., Severinsen, C., Kuehn, C., Straker, D., and Fritz, C.J. "Obstacles to Effective Case Mangement with AIDS Patients: The Clinician's Perspective," Social Work in Health Care, 1992, 17(2), 27-40.

* Wiener, L.S., and Siegel, K. "Social Workers' Comfort in Providing Services to AIDS Patients," Social Work, January 1990, 35, 18-25.

VIII. Services for the Elderly

* Burns, B.J., and Taube, C.A. "Mental Health Services in General Medical Care in Nursing Homes." In Fogel, B.S. et al. (eds.) Mental Health Policy for Older Americans: Protecting Minds at Risk. Washington DC:American Psychiatric Press, 1990.

* Generations, April 1990, XIV (2), 1-78. Special issue on Long-Term Care Financing.

* The Gerontologist. Special issue on "Ethnicity and Aging, Mental Health, Income and Demography," December 1990, 30(6).

* Kermis, M.D. Mental Health Late in Life, Chapter 1, "Concepts and Issues"; Chapter 4, "Stress and Social Adaptation"; and Chapter 10, "The Context of Care," Boston: Jones and Bartlett, 1986.

* Krause, N. "Social Supports, Stress, and Well-Being Among Older Adults," Journal of Gerontology, (41:4) 1986, 512-119.

* Kulys, R., and Davis, M.A. "An Analysis of Social Services in Hospices," Social Work, (31:6) November-December 1986, 448-455.

* Leutz, W., Abrahams, R., Greenlick, M., Kane, R., and Prottas, J. "Targeting Expanded Care to the Aged: Early HMO Experience," The Gerontological Society of America, (28:1) 1988, 4-17.

* Matlaw, J.R., and Mayer, J.B. "Elder Abuse: Ethical and Practice Dilemmas for Social Work," Health and Social Work, (11:2) Spring 1986, 85-94.

* Pillemer, K., and Finkelhor, D. "The Prevalence of Elder Abuse: A Random Sample Survey," The Gerontologist, (28:1) 1988, 51-57.

IX. Mental Health Policy and Programs

Historical Background; Legislation; Community Services; Deinstitutionalization

* Bachrach, L.L. "The Future of the State Mental Hospital," Hospital and Community Psychiatry, (37:5) May 1986, 467-474.

* Bloom, B. Community Mental Health: A General Introduction, Monterey, CA: Brooks/Cole, 1984, 1-65.

* Dumont, M.P. Treating the Poor. Belmont, MA: Dymphna Press, 1992.

* Feiner, J.S. "Both Ends of the River," Readings, March 1994, 9(1), 20-24. (RP) (This is a book review of Dumont's Treating the Poor).

* Goldman, H.H., and Morrissey, J.P. "The Alchemy of Mental Health Policy: Homelessness and the Fourth Cycle of Reform," American Journal of Public Health, (75:7) July 1985, 727-731.

* Johnson, A. B. Out of Bedlam: The Truth About Deinstitutionalization. New York: Basic Books, 1990.

* Mechanic, D. Mental Health and Social Policy, 3rd ed. Englewood Cliffs, NJ: Prentice Hall, 1989.

* Mechanic, D. "Mental Health Services in the Context of Health Insurance Reform," Milbank Quarterly, 1993, 71(3), 349-364.

* Mechanic, D. "Establishing Mental Health Priorities," Milbank Quarterly, 1994, 72(3), 501-514. (RP)

* Mechanic, D., Schlesinger, M., and McAlpine, D.D. "Management of Mental Health and Substance Abuse Services: State of the Art and Early Results," Milbank Quarterly, 1995, 73(1), 19-55. (RP)

X. Racism and Racial Issues

* Chung, H., Mahler, J.C., and Kakuma, T. "Racial Differences in Treatment of Psychiatric Inpatients," Psychiatric Services, June 1995, 46(6), 586-591. (RP)

* Wade, J.C. "Institutional Racism: An Analysis of the Mental Health System," American Journal of Orthopsychiatry, October 1993, 63(4), 536-544. (RP)

XI. Legal and Ethical Issues

* American Journal of Orthopsychiatry, special issue on legal issues in mental health, April 1994, volume 64(2).

* Wilk, R.J. "Are the Rights of People with Mental Illness Still Important?" Social Work, March 1994, 39(2), 167-175.

XII. Chronic (Severe and Persistent) Mental Illness

* Bachrach, L.L. "Defining Chronic Mental Illness: A Concept Paper," Hospital and Community Psychiatry, (39:4) April 1988, 383-388. (RP)

* Bachrach, L.L. "The Biopsychosocial Legacy," Hospital and Community Psychiatry, June 1993, 44(6),523-524. (RP)

* Bachrach, L.L. "Case Management: Toward a Shared Definition," Hospital and Community Psychiatry, Sept. 1989, 40, 883-884.

* Belcher, J.R. "The Trade-Offs of Developing a Case Management Model for Chronically Mentally Ill People," Health and Social Work, Feb. 1993, 18(1), 20-31. (RP)

* Brennan, J.P., and Kaplan, C. "Setting New Standards for Social Work Case Management," Hospital and Community Psychiatry, 1993, 44(3), 219-222.

* Freddolino, P.P. et al. "An Advocacy Model for People with Long-Term Psychiatric Disabilities," Hospital and Community Psychiatry, Nov. 1989, 40, 1169-1174.

* Koyanagi, C., and Goldman, H.H. "The Quiet Success of the National Plan for the Chronically Mentally Ill," Hospital and Community Psychiatry, 1991, 42(9), 899-905.

* Kruzich, J.M. The Chronically Mentally Ill in Nursing Homes: Issues in Policy and Practice," Health and Social Work, (11:1) Winter 1986, 5-13.

* Milbank Quarterly, 1994, volume 72(1), Providing Treatment to Persons with Mental Illness"—this is a special issue focused mainly on evaluations of the Robert Wood Johnson Foundation Program on Chronic Mental Illness.

* Munetz, M.R., Birnbaum, A., and Wyzik, P.F. "An Integrative Ideology to Guide Community-Based Multidisciplinary Care of Severely Mentally Ill Patients," Hospital and Community Psychiatry, June 1993, 44(6), 551-555.

* Rock, B.D., Haymes, E., Auerbach, C., Beckerman, A. "Helping Patients in the Supportive Milieu of a Community Residence Program for the Chronically Mentally Ill: Conceptual Model and Initial Evaluation," Social Work in Health Care, 1992, 16(3), 97-114.

* Rubin, A. "Is Case Management Effective for People with Serious Mental Illness? A Research Review" Health and Social Work, 1992, 17(2), 138-150.

* Swidler, R.N., and Tauriello, J.V. "New York State's Community Mental Health Reinvestment Act," Psychiatric Services, May 1995, 46(5), 496-500. (RP)

* Taube, C.A. et al. "New Directions in Research on Assertive Community Treatment," Hospital and Community Psychiatry, 1990, 41, 642-647.

* Thompson, K.S. et al. "A Historical Review of the Madison Model of Community Care," Hospital and Community Psychiatry, 1990, 41, 625-634.

* Torrey, E.F. "Economic Barriers to Widespread Implementation of Model Programs for the Seriously Mentally Ill," Hospital and Community Psychiatry, May 1990, 41, 526-531.

XIII. Homelessness and Mental Illness

* Bachrach, L.L. "What We Know About Homelessness Among Mentally Ill Persons: An Analytical Review and Commentary," Hospital and Community Psychiatry, 1992, 43(5), 453-464.

* Chandler, S.M. "Brown versus New York: The Rashomon of Delivering Mental Health Services in the 1990s," Health and Social Work, 1992, 17(2), 128-136.

* Cohen, N.L., Putnam, J.F., and Sullivan, A.M. "The Mentally Ill Homeless: Isolation and Adaptation," Hospital and Community Psychiatry, (35:9) September 1984, 922-924.

* Lamb, H.R. "Perspectives on Effective Advocacy for Homeless Mentally Ill Persons," Hospital and Community Psychiatry, 1992, 43(12), 1209-1212.

* Rife, J.C. et al. "Case Management with Homeless Mentally Ill People," Health and Social Work, 1991, 16(1), 58-67.(see also entire issue which is devoted to chronic mental illness)

XIV. Substance Abuse

* Buckner, J.C., and Mandell, W. "Risk Factors for Depressive Symptomatology in a Drug Using Population," American Journal of Public Health, May 1990, 80, 580-585.

* Feigelman, W. "Day Care Treatment for Multiple Drug Abusing Adolescents: Social Factors Linked with Completing Treatment," Journal of Psychoactive Drugs, (19:4) October-December 1987, 335-344.

* Hospital and Community Psychiatry, special issue on dual diagnoses of psychiatric and substance abuse syndromes, October 1989, 40(10), 1019-1049 (see articles by Lehman et al, Osher and Kofoed, Minkoff, Caton et al., Drake and Wallach; Thacker and Tremaine)

* The Milbank Quarterly. Confronting Drug Policy—Parts 1 and 2, special issue supplements, 1991, 69 (3&4).

XV. Program Evaluation and Research

Program Evaluation, Quality Assurance, Peer Review

* Berkman, B., and Rehr, H. "The Sick-Role Cycle and the Timing of Social Work Intervention," Social Service Review, 46, 1972, 567-580.

* Berkman, B. Bedell, D., Parker, E. et al. "Preadmission Screening: An Efficacy Study," Social Work in Health Care, (13:3) 1988, 35-50.

* Boone, C.R., Coulton, C.J., and Keller, S.M. "The Impact of Early and Comprehensive Social Work Services on Length of Stay," Social Work in Health Care, (7) Fall 1981, 1-9.

* Christ, W.R., Clarkin, J.F., and Hull, J.W. "A High-Risk Screen for Psychiatric Discharge Planning," Health and Social Work, Nov. 1994, 19(4), 261-270.

* Evans, R.L. et al. "Timing of Social Work Intervention and Medical Patients' Length of Hospital Stay," Health and Social Work, Nov. 1989, 14, 277-282.

* Hedblom, J.E., "Measuring Inpatient Psychosocial Severity: A Progress Report on the Development of an Instrument," Social Work in Health Care, (13:2) 1987, 59-73.

* Hsieh, M., and Kagle, J.D. "Understanding Patient Satisfaction and Dissatisfaction with Health Care," Health and Social Work, 1991, 16(4), 281-290.

* Rock, B. et al. "Psychosocial Factors as Predictors of Length of Stay for Medicare Patients Under the Prospective Payment System," Journal of Health and Social Policy, 1990, 2(2), 1-17.

* Vourlekis, B.S. "The Field's Evaluation of Proposed Clinical Indicators for Social Work Services in the Acute Care Hospital," Health and Social Work, Aug. 1990, 15(3), 197-206.

Research Issues and Approaches

* Berkman, B., and Weissman, L.A., "Applied Social Work Research," in R. Miller and H. Rehr (eds.), Social Work Issues in Health Care Practice. Englewood Cliffs, NJ: Prentice-Hall, 1983, 221-251.

* Bloom, B.L. "Assessing Community Structure and Community Need," pp. 355-392, in M. Bloom, Community Mental Health: A General Introduction. Monterey, CA: Brooks/Cole, 1984.

* Carlton, T.O., Flack, H.S., and Berkman, B. "The Use of Theoretical Constructs and Research Data to Establish a Base for Clinical Social Work in Health Settings," Social Work in Health Care, (10:2) Winter 1984, 27-40.

* Coulton, C.J. "Research and Practice: An Ongoing Relationship." Health and Social Work, (10:4) Fall 1985, 282-291. (RP)

* Gantt, A.B., and Levine, J. "The Roles of Social Work in Psycho-Biological Research," Social Work in Health Care, 1990, 15(2), 63-75.

* Roberts, C.S. et al. "Integrating Research with Practice: The Psychosocial Impact of Breast Cancer," Health and Social Work, Nov. 1989, 14(4), 261-268.

* Schaffer, M.A., and Lia-Hoagberg, B. "Prenatal Care Among Low-Income Women," Families in Society, March 1994, 152-159.

* Social Work in Health Care. Special issue on "Research Issues in Health Care Social Work," 1990, 15(1).

XVI. Health and Illness Behavior

Overview

* Bloom, B.L. "Basic Concepts in Prevention," pp. 191-243, in M. Bloom, Community Mental Health: A General Introduction. Monterey, CA: Brooks/Cole, 1984.

* Coulton, C. "Factors Related to Preventive Health Behavior: Implications for Social Work Intervention," Social Work in Health Care, (3) April 1978, 297-310. (RP)

* Freeman, H., and Levine, S. (eds., 4th edition), Handbook of Medical Sociology. Englewood Cliffs, NJ: Prentice Hall, 1989.

* Long, J.V.F., and Vaillant, G.E. "Natural History of Male Psychological Health, XI: Escape from the Underclass," American Journal of Psychiatry, (141:13) March 1984, 341- 346.

* Mechanic, D., Mental Health and Social Policy, Chapter 6.

* Mechanic, D., "Illness Behavior," Medical Sociology, New York: Free Press, 1978, 248- 289.

* Rosenberg, C.E. "Disease in History: Frames and Framers," Milbank Quarterly, 1989, 67(Supplement 1), 1-15.

* Zussman, R. "Life in the Hospital: A Review," Milbank Quarterly, 1993, 167-185.

Cross-Cultural Issues

* Gallegos, J.S. "Planning and Administering Services for Minority Groups," (Austin and Hershey, eds.), Handbook on Mental Health Administration, 87-105.

* Gil, R.M. "The Ethnic Patient: Implications for Medical Social Work Practice," Cross Cultural Issues: Impact on Social Work Practice in Health Care, Conference Proceedings, May 17, 1984, Columbia University School of Social Work (Maternal and Child Health Grant).

* Harwood, A. "Guidelines for Culturally Appropriate Health Care," in A. Harwood (ed.), Ethnicity and Medical Care, Cambridge, MA: Harvard University Press, 482-507. (Refer also to separate chapters on specific ethnic groups)

* Harwood, A. "The Hot-Cold Theory of Disease: Implications for Treatment of Puerto Rican Patients," Journal of the American Medical Association, May 17, 1971, 1153-1158.

* Jones, B.E., and Gray, B.A. "Problems in Diagnosing Schizophrenia and Affective Disorders Among Blacks," Hospital and Community Psychiatry, (37:1) January 1986, 61-65.

* Lawson, W.B. "Racial and Ethnic Factors in Psychiatric Research," Hospital and Community Psychiatry, (37:1) January 1986, 50-54.

* Payer, L. Medicine and Culture. New York: Penguin, 1988.

* Romanucci-Ross, The Anthropology of Medicine. New York: Bergin and Garvey, 1991.

* Waldfogel, S., and Wolpe, P.R. "Using Awareness of Religious Factors to Enhance Interventions in Consultation-Liaison Psychiatry," Hospital and Community Psychiatry, May 1993, 44(3), 473-477.

* Williams, D.H. "The Epidemiology of Mental Illness in Afro-Americans," Hospital and Community Psychiatry, (37:1) January 1986, 42-49.

XVII. Patient Rights; The Community and Self-Help; Partnerships between Professionals and Consumers

* Black, R.B., and Weiss, J.O. "Genetic Support Groups and Social Workers as Partners," Health and Social Work, May 1990, 15(2), 91-99.

* Caplan, G. Support Systems and Community Mental Health, New York: Behavioral Publications, 1974. (special emphasis on chapter 1)

* Delgado, M., and Humm-Delgado, D., "Natural Support Systems: Source of Strength in Hispanic Communities," Social Work, (27:1) January 1982, 83-89.

* Ell, K. "Social Networks, Social Support and Health Status: A Review," Social Service Review, March 1984, 133-147.

* Emerick, R.E. "Self-Help Groups for Former Patients; Relations with Mental Health Professionals," Hospital and Community Psychiatry, April 1990, 41, 401-407. (RP)

* Greenberg, J.S., Greenley, J.R., and Benedict, P. "Contributions of Persons with Serious Mental Illness to their Families," Hospital and Community Psychiatry, May 1994, 45(5), 475-480.

* Grosser, R.C., and Vine, P. "Families as Advocates for the Mentally Ill: A Survey of Characteristics and Service Needs," American Journal of Orthopsychiatry, April 1991, 61(2), 282-290.

* Hardt, B., and Halkin, K.R. The New Way to Take Charge of your Medical Treatment: A Patient's Guide. New York: Madison Books.

* Kelley, P., and Kelley, V.R. "Supporting Natural Helpers: A Cross-Cultural Study," Social Casework, (66:6) June 1985, 358-366.

* Kurtz, L.F., and Chambon, A. "Comparison of Self-Help Groups for Mental Health," Health and Social Work, (12:4) Fall 1987, 275-283. (RP)

* Levin, L., and Idler, E.L., The Hidden Health Care System: Mediating Structures and Medicine, Cambridge, MA: Ballinger, 1981; Ch. 2, "Families and Self-Care," 55-111; Ch. 4, "Community Groups and Mutual Aid," 159-184.

* Lurie, A., and Shulman, L. "The Professional Connection with Self-Help Groups in Health Care Settings," Social Work in Health Care, (8:4) Summer 1983, 69-77.

* Mayer, J.B. et al. "Empowering Families of the Chronically Ill: A Partnership Experience in a Hospital Setting," Social Work in Health Care, 1990, 14(4), 73-90.

* Powell, T.J. Self-Help Organizations and Professional Practice. Washington, DC: NASW, 1987.

* Powell, T.J. Working with Self-Help. Washington DC: NASW, 1990.

* Rehr, H. "The Consumer and Consumerism," in R. Miller and H. Rehr (eds.), Social Work Issues in Health Care Practice. Englewood Cliffs, NJ: Prentice-Hall, 1983, 20-73.

* Riessman, F., and Carroll, D. Redefining Self-Help: Policy and Practice. San Francisco: Jossey-Bass, 1995.

* Simonson, S.K. "Peer Counseling in Health Care: A Collaboration of Social Work and Voluntarism," Social Work in Health Care, (12:4) Summer 1987, 1-19.

* Soskis, C.W., and Kerson, T.S. "The Patient Self Determination Act: Opportunity Knocks Again," Social Work in Health Care, 1992, 16(4). 1-18.

XVIII. Professional Issues for Social Workers in Health

Interdisciplinary Collaboration

* Abramson, J., and Mizrahi, T. "Strategies for Enhancing Collaboration Between Social Workers and Physicians," Social Work in Health Care, (12:1) Fall 1986, 1-21. (RP)

* Berger, C.S. "Enhancing Social Work Infuence in the Hospital: Identifying Sources of Power," Social Work in Health Care, 1990, 15(2), 77-93.

* Connaway, R.S. "Teamwork and Social Worker Advocacy: Conflicts and Possibilities." Community Mental Health Journal, (11:4) 1975, 381-388.

* Dana, B. "The Collaborative Process," in R. Miller and H. Rehr (eds.), Social Work Issues in Health Care Practice. Englewood Cliffs, NJ: Prentice-Hall, 1983, 181-220.

* Davidson, K.W. "Role Blurring and the Hospital Social Worker's Search for a Clear Domain," Health and Social Work, August 1990, 15(3), 228-234.

* Mailick, M., and Ashley, "Interprofessional Collaboration, Challenge to Advocacy," Social Casework, 62, 1981, 131-137.

* Mizrahi, T., and Abramson, J. "Sources of Strain Between Physicians and Social Workers: Implications for Social Workers in Health Care Settings," Social Work in Health Care, (10:3) Spring 1985, 33-51. (RP)

* Roberts, C.S. "Conflicting Professional Values in Social Work and Medicine," Health and Social Work, 1989, 14(3), 211-218. (RP)

* Schuster, J.M., Kern, E.E., Kane, V., and Nettleman, L. "Changing Roles of Mental Health Clinicians in Multidisciplinary Teams," Hospital and Community Psychiatry, December 1994, 45(12), 1187-1189. (RP)

* Toseland, R.W. et al. "Teamwork in Psychiatric Settings," Social Work, 1986, 31(1), 46-52.

Discharge Planning

* Caputi, M.A., and Heiss, W.A. "The DRG Revolution," Health and Social Work, (9:1) Winter , 1984, 5-12.

* Dobrof, J. "DRGs and the Social Worker's Role in Discharge Planning," Social Work in Health Care, 1991, 16(2), 37-54. (RP)

* Marcus, L.J. "Discharge Planning: An Organizational Perspective," Health and Social Work, Winter 1987, 39-45.

* Wolock, I., Schlesinger, E., Dinerman, M., and Seaton, R., "The Posthospital Needs and Care of Patients: Implications for Discharge Planning," Social Work in Health Care, (12:4) Summer 1987, 61-76.

Ethics and Values

* Abramson, M. "Ethics and Technological Advances: Contributions of Social Work Practice," Social Work in Health Care, 1990, 15(2), 5-17. (RP)

* Bahou, C., and Gralnick, M. "High-Risk Conversations: A Response to Reamer," Social Work, May 1989, 34(3), 262-264.

* Bayer, R., Callahan, D., Caplan, A.L., and Jennings, B. "Toward Justice in Health Care," American Journal of Public Health, (78:5) May 1988, 583-588.

* Blumenfield, S., and Lowe, J.I. " A Template for Analyzing Ethical Dilemmas in Discharge Planning," Health and Social Work, Winter 1987, 12(1), 47-56.

* Callahan, D. Setting Limits: Medical Goals in Aging Society. New York: Touchstone, 1987.

* Callahan, D. "Reforming the Health Care System for Children and the Elderly to Balance Cure and Care," Academic Medicine, April 1992, 67(4), 219-222. (RP)

* Daniels, N. "Why Saying No to Patients in the United States is So Hard: Cost Containment, Justice and Provider Autonomy," New England Journal of Medicine, 1986, 314, 1381-1383.

* Furlong, R., "The Social Worker's Role on the Institutional Ethics Committee," Social Work in Health Care, (II:4) Summer 1986, 93-100.

* Loewenberg, F.M., and Dolgoff, R. Ethical Decisions for Social Work Practice, 4th ed. Itasca, IL: F.E. Peacock, 1992.

* National Association of Social Workers, "Client Self-Determination in End-Of-Life Decisions." Statement adopted by the NASW Delegate Assembly, 1993.

* Orentlicher, D. "The Right to Die After Cruzan," Journal of the American Medical Association, November 14, 1990, 264(18), 2444-2446.

* Proctor, E.K., Morrow-Howell, N., and Lott, C.L. "Classification and Correlates of Ethical Dilemmas in Hospital Social Work," Social Work, March 1993, 38(2), 166-177.

* Reamer, F. "The Emergence of Bioethics in Social Work," Health and Social Work, 1985, 10, 271-288.

* Reamer, F.G. "Aids and Ethics: The Agenda for Social Workers," Social Work, Sept.-Oct. 1988, 5, 460-464.

* Wilk, R.J. "Are the Rights of People with Mental Illness Still Important?" Social Work, March 1994, 39(2), 167-175.

XIX. Conclusions and Future Perspectives

* Dillon, C. "Managing Stress in Health Social Work Roles Today," Social Work in Health Care, 1990, 14(11), 91-108.

* Sabin, J.E. "Clinical Skills for the 1990s: Six Lessons from HMO Practice," Hospital and Community Psychiatry, 1991, 42(6), 605-608. (RP)

* Schreter, R.K. "Ten Trends in Managed Care and Their Impact on the Biopsychosocial Model," Hospital and Community Psychiatry, April 1993, 44(4), 325-327.

APPENDIX ONE—USEFUL WEB LINKS

Government Sites

*   Agency for Health Care Policy and Research, http://www.ahcpr.gov/

    "AHCPR, a part of the U.S. Department of Health and Human Services, is the lead agency charged with supporting research designed to improve the quality of health care, reduce its cost, and broaden access to essential services."

*   Department of Health & Human Services, http://www.hhs.gov/

    The federal agency responsible for "protecting the health of all Americans and providing essential human services, especially for those who are least able to help themselves."

*   Health Care Financing Administration, http://www.hcfa.gov/

    Federal agency that administers the Medicare, Medicaid and Child Health Insurance programs.

*   healthfinder™, http://www.healthfinder.gov/

    "healthfinder™ is a gateway consumer health and human services information website from the United States government. Healthfinder™ can lead you to selected online publications, clearinghouses, databases, websites, and support and self-help groups, as well as the government agencies and not-for-profit organizations that produce reliable information for the public....The healthfinder™ website has been developed by the Department of Health and Human Services (HHS), in collaboration with other federal agencies. The project is coordinated by the Office of Disease Prevention and Health Promotion (ODPHP), with the active participation of a Steering Committee composed of representatives of the federal agencies whose information is included in healthfinder™ and non-federal consumer health information specialists, librarians, and others actively engaged in the provision or use of online consumer health information. Significant support for the project is provided by the National Health Information Center."

*   Social Security Online, http://www.ssa.gov/

    The official website of the Social Security Administration.

*   Thomas: Legislative Information on the Internet, http://thomas.loc.gov/

    Maintained by the Library of Congress, Thomas (after Thomas Jefferson) includes the full-text of U.S. public bills and laws, the Congressional Record and Index, and committee reports.

Non-Governmental Organizations/Websites

*   The Alpha Center, http://www.ac.org/

    "Established in 1976, this non-profit and non-partisan health policy center helps public and private sector clients respond to health care challenges by providing the essential keys to policy-making: objective information, insightful analysis, and expert strategic planning and program management." Includes an extensive list of web links to health care policy resources.

*   American Herbal Products Association, http://www.ahpa.org/

    "The national trade association and voice of the herbal and herbal products industry."

*   NHeLP: National Health Law Program, Inc., http://www.healthlaw.org/

    "The National Health Law Program is a national public interest law firm that seeks to improve health care for America's working and unemployed poor, minorities, the elderly and people with disabilities. NHeLP serves legal services programs, community-based organizations, the private bar, providers and individuals who work to preserve a health care safety net for the millions of uninsured or underinsured low-income people."

*   The Urban Institute, http://www.urban.org/

    "A nonpartisan economic, social, and policy research organization. The Urban Institute investigates social and economic problems confronting the nation and analyzes efforts to solve these problems. The Institute seeks to increase Americans' awareness of important public choices and improve the formulation and implementation of government decisions. Much of its research is available to the public." Site includes a wealth of information on U.S. health care policy and research.

Web Guides

* The Alternative Medicine HomePage, http://www.pitt.edu/~cbw/altm.html

   "The Alternative Medicine HomePage is a jumpstation for sources of information on unconventional, unorthodox, unproven, or alternative, complementary, innovative, integrative therapies." Includes links to Internet resources, mailing lists and newsgroups, and government resources.

* Emory University Health Sciences Center Library: MedWeb, http://www.gen.emory.edu/medweb/

   An extensive, lightly annotated collection of medicine-related sites. In particular, see the entries on Health Care Reform and Bioethics.

* Health Law Hippo, http://hippo.findlaw.com/

   "Health Hippo is a collection of policy and regulatory materials related to health care, with some graphics sprinkled in." See especially Health Hippo: Policy and Administration, which includes links to recent legislation/testimony, news, and related websites.

* @Inside Health Care Website, http://www.InsideHealthCare.com/

   An extensive list of health care sites; includes a section on policy sites.

* National Institutes of Health Library—Internet Sites, http://libwww.ncrr.nih.gov/sitesindex.htm

   See in particular the Statistics entry under the Reference Resources section.

* Yahoo!, Internet search engine's category listings:

   Health: Health Care, http://www.yahoo.com/Health/Health_Care/

   Health: Health Care: Policy, http://www.yahoo.com/Health/Health_Care/Policy/

Bulletin Board

A web-based bulletin board, known as a CUBboard (for "Columbia University Bulletin Board"), has been created for this class. The board may be used for announcements, queries, and discussion. Please check the board periodically for messages by visiting the following web page:

   https://www1.columbia.edu/sec/bboard/983/socw6910-001/index.html *[Editor's note: password protected.]*

Access to the board is limited to students registered for T6910, and the instructors. You will be asked to enter your cunix e-mail ID and password to confirm your identity.

APPENDIX TWO—IN-CLASS EXERCISES AND HANDOUTS

Public Care Policy Exercise (Session 1)

Health care policy is not made arbitrarily, but rather is constructed by answering some fundamental questions regarding our value system. The aim of their exercise is to evaluate the values embedded in our current health policies and its consequences.

Your instructor will assign you to a small work group. Each work group will examine the values/principles that guide our current health care system using the following values/principles as a guideline:

* Consumer Choice (full choice, limited choice, or no choice)

* Equal rights? (e.g., Is health care a right? If yes, should everyone get the same level of services?)

* Communal/societal responsibilities

* Efficiency and cost (e.g., Should individual contribution be aligned with individual benefits?)

Using the above guideline, each group should spend 20–30 minutes developing a statement that answers the following questions:

1. What are the dominant values/principles that exist in our current health care system?

2. What are the consequences of those values?

3. In your group's opinion, are the values/principles listed for your group ideal? If yes, why? If no, why?

At the end of this time, each group will report to the class their findings and evaluations.

Health Care Policy Exercise (Session 2)

In recent years, federal and state governments have embraced managed care as their solution to escalating health care costs and to mend our fragmented health care system. In 1997, Medicare instituted Medicare Choice and many states have mandated Medicaid recipients to join HMOs. Today's exercise is designed to help social work students to critically think about managed care system in public programs.

Your instructor will assign you to small work groups (see below). Groups with a "pro" platform will argue for managed care systems and its implication for financing, policy and care. Groups with a "con" platform will argue against managed care systems and its implications for financing, policy and care.

	Managed Medicare	Managed Medicaid
Pro	A	B
Con	C	D

Each group will have 30 minutes to prepare a statement that answers the following questions:

1. What population does managed Medicare/Medicaid serve?

2. What are the advantages/disadvantages of managed care for the population served in each program? (Examine issues of access to care, efficiency, quality of care).

3. What role should social workers have within managed care organizations?

After the 30-minute small-group discussion session, each group is expected to present their position to class (5–8 minutes per group).

Workshop on Diversity and Mental Health (Session 5)

For this workshop read the required and recommended reading material. Come to class prepared to report and discuss your experience providing Social Work services to people of a diverse group, different than your own.

Divide into small working groups. Each group should have no more than six and no fewer than three members. These groups will have 20–30 minutes to share and discuss with each other their experiences of providing social work services in the health system. There are no definite questions to address, however, groups should take into consideration the following:

1. Identify the values expressed by your client group regarding health and mental health issues.

2. What were, if any, the difficulties due to cultural differences that you experienced in providing social work services.

3. What were, if any, the difficulties stemming from the structure, policies, access, and location of your agency that interfered with serving the client group.

4. Identify the perspectives, attitudes, and expectations of your client group towards health care providers (doctors, nurses, social workers, etc.)

5. Identify this group's understanding, attitudes, acceptance, refusal to differential diagnosis, and treatment.

In conclusion each group will be asked to make a brief (no more than 5 minutes) presentation of the key issues in providing Health/Mental Health services to these diverse groups. Questions, comments, and examples will be encouraged

Health Care Policy Exercise: Developmental Issues (Session 12)

Social attitudes towards, and personal experience with, different age groups affect how society decides to allocate health care resources. The aim of this exercise is to examine this premise and to see consequences regarding social work advocacy.

Each student determines a favored population to work with. Students should form small groups according to population of preference. (For example, all interested in working with adolescence, get into the same group.)

Once groupings are completed, switch half the groups' assignments. Give to one half of the groups a completely different assigned population as a focus. (For example, people with declared interest in adolescence, now must work with the aged)

Next, have all groups develop a policy for their patient population. Chronic mental health might be a subject for this policy.

Groups then feed back their experiences to the whole class according to the following guidelines:

1. What assumptions did students make while developing the policy which might have been based on their understanding of the developmental, biological, social, and psychological signposts of their populations?

2. What implications did their understanding of developmental issues have for their policy development and formulation? To be included here is the implication for social work advocacy practice.

Public Health and Research (Session 13)

1. Articulate a public health problem that has implications for health policy.

2. Discuss why this is a public health problem and why social work intervention is appropriate.

3. Identify and briefly discuss a level of intervention you would propose using to address the problem.

4. What data would you need in order to determine the a) scope of the problem, b) the etiology of the problem, and c) possible interviews strategy(ies).

APPENDIX THREE—RESEARCH AIDS

Researching Health Policy Legislation

This is a brief guide to researching current health policy issues and legislation in the U.S. on the internet. Keyword and subject searches on CLIO (http://www.columbia.edu/cu/libraries/clio_plus) will locate relevant government documents in the Documents Service Center (DSC). All DSC items are located in the East Reading Room of Lehman Library. Note: The CLIO record will not tell you if the item is in microfiche! You should check both the print stacks and the microfiche cabinets, using the call number on CLIO.

Access Restrictions: available to current Columbia faculty, staff and students only.

Tracking legislation through Congress can be a complicated process. Consult the DSC guide, *The Legislative Process*, for a step-by-step explanation of the process and the tools, both in print and on the internet, used for following legislation from the introduction of a bill, to its passage into law, to eventual regulatory enforcement.

Another web page, designed for the SIPA Health Policy concentration, may also be of use. It concentrates on U.S. executive agency and state internet sites.

Sources for Legislation and Policy

The major U.S. governmental sites for health policy legislation are:

* *Major Legislation by Topic, 105th Congress,* from Thomas website.

   Click on "health policy" to retrieve a list of bills that relate to that topic. The same option is available for the 104th Congress. You can also do a phrase search on a more specific topic, such as "home health" at the main Thomas web page.

* *Bills, Laws, and Regulations,* from Congressional Universe website, http://www.library.yale.edu/pubstation/databases/congressional.html

   Each can be searched by keyword, or by bill number (back to 1989), P.L. number (back to 1989), or FR/CFR citation (current). You can also search CIS Legislative Histories by keyword back to 1970. Legislative Histories are the detailed records of congressional legislation, containing references to all bills, hearings, committee reports, etc., associated with all public laws.

   The print version of Congressional Universe is the CIS Index, located on the Lehman Reference Index Tables. It can be more efficient to consult the printed indexes for older material, since there are legislative histories compiled for laws passed since 1970.

* *Health Care Financing Administration (HCFA)* website.

   HCFA is the federal agency that administers the Medicare, Medicaid and Child Health Insurance Programs. Much information is available on this site, including health care spending projections, the Medicare Handbook, statistics and data, etc. Of particular interest is the section on Laws & Regulations, which contains links to full text of major legislation affecting HCFA, the President's legislative proposals, hearings and appeals, and Federal Register notices.

* *Office of Management and Budget (OMB)* website, http://www.whitehouse.gov/WH/EOP/OMB/html/ombhome.html

   OMB's predominant mission is to assist the president in overseeing the preparation of the federal budget and to supervise its administration in executive branch agencies. In helping to formulate the president's spending plans, OMB evaluates the effectiveness of agency programs, policies, and procedures, assesses competing funding demands among agencies, and sets funding priorities. OMB ensures that agency reports, rules, testimony, and proposed legislation are consistent with the president's budget and with administration policies.

   Under "Legislative Information," there are two useful sections:

   * Statements of Administration Policy: provides official White House policy on bills before Congress.
   * Agencies' Communications to Congress: provides text of each agencies' Congressional testimony, often in relation to bills in committee or on the floor of Congress.

* *President's Advisory Commission on Consumer Protection and Quality in the Health Care Industry*

   The commission was created by President Clinton to "advise the President on changes occurring in the health care system and recommend such measures as may be necessary to promote and assure health care quality and value, and protect consumers and workers in the health care system." Includes the Consumer Bill of Rights and Responsibilities and the Commission's final report, Quality First: Better Health Care for All Americans, released March 12, 1998.

Background Information & Evaluation in Journals

Sources for background information on legislation, its implementation, and consequences are:

- *Congressional Quarterly Weekly Report.* Washington, DC: Congressional Quarterly.

- *Congressional Quarterly Almanac.* Annual. Washington, DC: CQ Press.

  CQ covers everything that goes on in Congress, indexed; useful to determine dates, chronologies, bill titles and numbers. Also a good source for a succinct analysis of the issues related to a particular piece of legislation. Use the weeklies for current legislation, the annual almanac for prior years.

- *Health Care Financing Review.* Quarterly. Washington, DC: Health Care Financing Administration

  Scholarly journal from HCFA—a good source for comprehensive health care financing information, including evaluation and review. Not indexed in Social Work Abstracts (see below).

- *Lexis-Nexis Academic Universe.*

  A source of full text newspapers and news magazines; useful for reportage and public debate of issues.

- Social Work Abstracts (SWAB). Monthly. Washington, DC: NASW Press.

  SWAB is the index to journal literature in the field of social work. It can be supplemented by journal literature searches in some more general, or related indexes, such as Child Development Abstracts, ERIC, PsycInfo, Social Sciences Abstracts, Sociological Abstracts, etc. Ask a reference librarian for relevant indexes to your topic.

Sources for Evaluation within Government

Evaluation of legislation within the government can take place in a number of places, for a variety of reasons. Within the agency most concerned with the legislation, there may be followup studies, additional research, Congressional testimony, etc. The agency web page is a good place to start— look for terms like testimony, policy, research, evaluations, communications to Congress, etc.

There are some agencies which exist solely to serve as "watchdogs" of other agencies and their expenditures and policies. They are:

- Congressional Budget Office (CBO)

  CBO's mission is to provide the Congress with objective, timely, nonpartisan analyses needed for economic and budget decisions and with the information and estimates required for the Congressional budget process. Types of documents to be found here are: studies and reports, cost estimates, and testimony.

- FinanceNet

  The mission of FinanceNet is to "improve accountability and stewardship of public financial assets."

  One of the areas in the U.S. Federal section of FinanceNet is Major Documents. The types of documents available here are: accountability reports, annual reports, budgets, financial statements, five-year plans, performance agreements, performance plans, and strategic plans.

- General Accounting Office (GAO)

  GAO is the investigative arm of Congress. Charged with examining matters relating to the receipt and disbursement of public funds, GAO performs audits and evaluations of Government programs and activities. Go to "GAO Reports and Testimony." There are options to look at Reports and Testimony Issued since July 1, 1998, by title or by subject, and Reports and Testimony FY 1995–present.

University of North Carolina at Chapel Hill
School of Social Work

Course Title: Health, Illness, and Disability (SoWo 237)
Fall 1998

Course Instructor: Kathleen A. Rounds

DESCRIPTION

This course examines the psychosocial and biological determinants of health, illness, and disability across the life cycle. The main focus concerns the impact of illness and disability on individual development and family functioning.

OBJECTIVES

Upon completion of the course, students should be able to:

1. Define health, illness, and sick role behavior.
2. Identify the major determinants of health and illness (e.g., gender, race, socioeconomic status, environment, health behavior).
3. Describe the relationship between stress and health/illness and the factors that modify this relationship.
4. Demonstrate knowledge of the factors that influence health and illness behavior and health-related decisions.
5. Identify major health problems that disrupt development at each stage of the life cycle and examine their impact on individual development and family functioning.
6. Describe how an individual's/family's developmental stage influences the ability to understand and cope with illness and disability.
7. Demonstrate knowledge and understanding of loss/grief theories and the biopsychosocial impact of anticipatory grief, death, and bereavement on individuals and families.

TEXTS

Required Readings

A course pack including most of the required readings will be available from UNC Student Stores. An asterisk indicates that the assigned reading is *not included* in the coursepack due to copyright restrictions/excessive cost. All readings with an * are in the Social Work Resource Room.

Optional Texts

Biegel, D., Sales, E., & Schulz, R. (1991). *Family caregiving in chronic illness: Alzheimer's disease, cancer, heart disease, mental illness and stroke.* Newbury Park, CA: Sage.

Ell, K., & Northen, H. (1990). *Families and health care: Psychosocial practice.* New York: Aldine de Gruyter.

Rolland, J.S. (1994). *Families, illness, and disability.* New York: Basic Books.

COURSE REQUIREMENTS

I. This course will be conducted as a seminar to facilitate student participation. You are expected to read all assigned material prior to class and actively participate in class discussions. A small group of students will facilitate discussions of the assigned readings for each session (a sign-up sheet will be circulated at the first class session). Class attendance is essential—if you cannot attend, please notify the instructor.

A Listserv for this course will be available to encourage e-mail discussions among course members. This will be a closed list; access will be restricted to members of the course. You are required to participate in the Listserv at least three times during the semester.

II. The three main assignments are:

1. Ethnographic Interview. Due Session 7 at the beginning of class. This assignment is designed to help you understand the experience and perspective of an individual (or of a caregiver) who is living with an illness, disability, or health problem. See description below for specific guidelines.

2. Group Presentation. To be scheduled. This assignment gives you the opportunity to educate your colleagues about an illness, disability, or health problem of compelling interest to you, and to illustrate how it affects individual development and family functioning. See description for specific guidelines.

3. Final Exam. Due December 7th by 5:00 p.m. This "take home" essay exam will be available on Session 15 and will cover material from the entire semester including lectures, readings, classroom discussions, guest speaker topics, and videotapes.

Student learning will be evaluated by and grades will be based on:

Class Participation	10%
Interview Assignment	30%
Group Presentation	25%
Final Exam	35%

HONOR CODE

The Honor Code is in effect in this course. The following are my expectations in terms of Honor Code standards regarding assignments for this course:

Ethnographic Interview: You may consult with others prior to conducting your interview. However, your summary and critique of the interview must be completed without assistance from others.

Class Presentation: You are encouraged to consult with others outside your group to prepare this presentation. The bibliography should be prepared only by members of your group and should include only materials with which you are familiar. The source of all overheads that you use and handouts that you distribute in class should be cited on the material.

Final Exam: This is a take-home, open book exam. You may use any materials from the course, but may not consult with others. Give complete citations for ideas that are not your own. Please attach a sheet of paper on which you have written and signed the honor code pledge.

ASSIGNMENT 1—ETHNOGRAPHIC INTERVIEW

Objective

To understand what it means to "live with" a chronic/serious illness from a person who has an illness, or is the primary caregiver of someone who has a chronic/serious illness or disability.

In general, social scientists rely on two perspectives to study the illness experience: outsiders' and insiders' perspectives. The majority of assigned readings for this class were written from an outsider's perspective, which is based on medical, psychological, and sociological theories that emphasize deductive (hypothesis testing) processes. In contrast, an insider's perspective is primarily an inductive process that focuses on "the subjective experience of living with and in spite of illness" (Roth, J.A., & Conrad, P. [1987]. *Research in the sociology of health care.* Greenwich, CT: JAI Press, p. 2). One way to adopt an insider's perspective is to conduct an ethnographic interview using the guidelines specified below.

Guidelines

1. Select an informant who is *not* related to you and is currently experiencing a chronic/serious illness or disability, or is the primary caregiver, relative, or significant other of someone who has a chronic/serious illness or disability.

2. The major objective of the interview is to gain an insider's view of the informant's experience of living with a chronic/serious illness, disability, or health crisis. Since informants are living day-to-day with their condition, they are considered the "experts," and you should approach them with a posture of naive ignorance. You should assume the role of student-learner and ask the informant to teach you about his/her experience and to identify what he/she thinks is important for you to learn about daily life as a person who is living with cancer, cardiac disease, HIV, cystic fibrosis, etc.

3. Unlike a clinical interview, which focuses on assessment and intervention strategies, the ethnographic interview approach focuses on three main dimensions: (1) the meaning of the illness; (2) the types of strategies used to cope with the illness; and (3) the way in which the person organizes his/her world in the context of illness.

4. Interviews should be approximately 40–60 minutes long and may be tape-recorded (with the informant's permission) or recorded by taking detailed handwritten notes during the session. The interview should be fairly open, yet focused enough so that you can develop an understanding of what it's like to live with that person's illness/disability/health crisis. Confidentiality must be upheld and discussed with the informant before the interview occurs.

5. Develop an interview guide to refer to during your interview. The following are suggestions for what you might cover:
   - how the person first noticed that something was wrong
   - initial feelings/response to symptoms and/or diagnosis, and what it meant for that person
   - what brought the person in to seek help and what were primary concerns, fears, worries
   - how the person made sense of his/her illness, disability, health crisis (i.e., what kinds of explanations/theories about "why me?")
   - how the person's culture, ethnicity, or philosophical or religious beliefs has affected the illness experience
   - how he/she copes with the illness, disability, and/or health crisis on a daily basis
   - impact of illness and treatment on self, family life, work, career plans, social relationships, etc.
   - access to health care and interactions with health care providers

6. Summarize your interview in 3–5 double-spaced, typed pages (removing all identifying names), including at least 3 direct quotes from the informant. Also, provide a 2–3 page critique of your interview, addressing *all* the questions below:

    a. In general, how well do you think you elicited information from the informant about his/her illness experience/role as caregiver?

    b. Name two things you might have done differently in the interview and explain why.

    c. Looking back, what areas do you wish you had covered in the interview but did not? Explain.

    d. How "connected" did you feel to the informant and why, and what part of the interview was most difficult for you to "stay with" and why?

    e. What was the most compelling thing you learned about the informant/caregiver's experience from an insider's perspective? Additional comments?

7. Attach your interview guide.

Please type your Personal Identification Number at the top right hand corner of each page;
do not include your name.

ASSIGNMENT 2—GROUP PRESENTATION

1. I recommend that you select a topic for which you have a deep concern or commitment. Think in terms of your field placement or future career objectives. How can you structure this presentation so that it will have considerable relevance to your field placement and/or career objectives? Use this as an opportunity to explore a health problem or issue that you always wanted to know about, but haven't had the chance to examine in depth.

2. How should the presentation relate to the material discussed in class? I would like to see you bring relevant course material to bear on your topic in a creative way. For example, you could apply a model that explains the relationship between stress and disease outcomes to recovery from cancer.

3. Your presentation should include (if relevant), but is not limited to, the following:

    a. Description of the health problem: definition, incidence, and/or prevalence in the general population; population groups that are most affected (gender, age, ethnic minority, economic class, etc.) and why; etiology of the problem (biopsychosocial factors that contribute to the problem); association with other diseases; and prognosis.

    b. Issues regarding primary and secondary prevention.

    c. Issues surrounding treatment (types of treatment available, side effects from treatment, access and cost of treatment, treatment decision making, ethical issues regarding treatment).

    d. Impact of the problem on the individual's development. If the health problem only occurs during a specific developmental stage, then discuss its impact on development during that particular stage of the life cycle; otherwise, discuss its impact on human development throughout the life cycle. You may choose to limit your topic, for example, "The Effects of Diabetes on Adolescent Development." Or you can approach it more broadly, for example, "The Effects of Diabetes on Human Development Throughout the Life Cycle." Also, address how development affects the way in which individuals deal with this health problem.

    e. Impact of the health problem on the family or larger social network. Address how the family's developmental stage affects illness management. In some cases it may be relevant to discuss the impact of the health problem on the community, for example, "The impact of HIV disease on specific communities."

    f. Other psychosocial issues related to the health problem.

    g. Legal issues related to the health problem.

h. Implications for social work intervention; however, this should not be the main focus of the presentation.

4. The presentation should be more than just descriptive, reflecting your own thinking and critical analysis.

5. At the time of your presentation, hand out an outline and list of references to all class members. Include at least three references from the Internet. Also, feel free to use any audio visual materials if these would add to your presentation. Notify me several weeks in advance if you need other equipment than a VCR.

6. Since most of you will be doing your presentation as part of a small group, I will give you a group grade. If you wish to be graded individually, speak with me prior to your presentation.

General Grading Criteria for Presentation

1. Content: relevant, thorough, current
2. Organization: well organized, coherent, not repetitious, flows well; coordination of presentation among group members
3. Effectiveness of presentation: material presented in an interesting, engaging, and clear manner; effective use and integration of visual and oral presentation materials

COURSE OUTLINE

Session 1   Course Introduction
Session 2   Epidemiology of Health and Disease
Session 3   The Genetic Base (Guest Speaker)
Session 4   Health Behavior / Stress and Illness
Session 5   Family Systems, Illness, and Disability
Session 6   Prenatal Development and Infancy
Session 7   Preschool / School Age Child
             Interview Assignment due
Session 8   Adolescence
Session 9   Student Presentations
Session 10   Young Adulthood
Session 11   Student Presentations
Session 12   Middle Adult Years
Session 13   Student Presentations
Session 14   Older Adulthood
Session 15   Older Adulthood
             Distribute Final Exam
Session 16   Death and Bereavement
*** Final Exam Due December 7th by 5:00 p.m. ***

REQUIRED READINGS AND INTERNET RESOURCES

Session 1—Course Introduction

Session 2—Epidemiology of Health and Disease

Total Readings: 56 pages

Ness, R.B., & Kuller, L.M. (1997). Women's health as a paradigm for understanding factors that mediate disease. *Journal of Women's Health, 6*(3), 329-336. (8 pgs.)

*Northridge, M.E., & Shepard, P.M. (1997). Comment: Environmental racism and public health. *American Journal of Public Health, 87*(5), 730-732. (3)

Paulozzi, L.J., Keenan, N.L., & Truman, B.I. (1994). *Chronic Disease in Minority Populations,* (pp. 6.1-6.7). Atlanta: Centers for Disease Control. (7)

Williams, D.R., & Collins, C. (1995). U.S. socioeconomic and racial differences in health: Patterns and explanations. *Annual Review of Sociology, 27,* 349-386. (38)

Web Sites

Centers for Disease Control and Prevention, http://www.cdc.gov/ For more specifics, try http://www.cdc.gov/diseases/diseases.html

Center on Access to Disability Data, http://www.infouse.com/disabilitydata/index.html

Combined Health Information Database (CHID), http://chid.nih.gov/index.html

Health A to Z—Women's Health, http://www.HealthAtoZ.com/categories/WH.htm

Healthfinder (DHHS), http://www.healthfinder.org/default.htm This site, maintained by the U.S. Department of Health and Human Services, is the most comprehensive health-related website. It includes links and information about virtually any question related to public health or health conditions. Many of the more specific sites were links from Healthfinder.

Jacobs Institute of Women's Health, http://www.jiwh.org/

Minority Health Project, http://www.minority.unc.edu

The New York Times Women's Health Page, http://www.nytimes.com/women/

Office of Minority Health Resource Center, http://www.omhrc.gov/frames.htm

Women's Health: the Public Health Service Agenda, http://www.inform.umd.edu/EdRes/Topic/WomensStudies/GenderIssues/WomensHealth/phs-agenda This page is maintained by the University of Maryland, and has numerous informative links.

Women's Health America Group, http://www2.womenshealth.com/~wha/

Session 3—The Genetic Base

Total Readings: 96 pages + 1 article

Bernhardt, B., & Rauch, J.B. (1993). Genetic family histories: An aid to social work assessment. *Families in Society, 74*(4), 195-205. (11)

*Rauch, J.B., & Black, R.B. (1990). Genetics. In R.L. Edwards (Ed.-in-Chief), *Encyclopedia of social work,* (19th ed., pp. 1108-1116). Washington, DC: NASW Press. (9)

*Rothenberg, K. (1994). *Women and prenatal testing: Facing the challenge of genetic technology.* (Chapters 11-14; pp. 219-294). (76) [peruse]

Read one article from the following selection and use the Listserv to discuss:

*Carmi, R. (1991, Feb. 2). Genetic counseling to a traditional society. *The Lancet, 337,* p. 306. (1)

*Hill, S. (1994). Motherhood and the obfuscation of medical knowledge: The case of sickle cell disease. *Gender and Society, 8*(1), 29-47. (19)

*Neal-Cooper, F., & Scott, R.B. (1988). Genetic counseling in sickle cell anemia: Experiences with couples at risk. *Public Health Reports, 103*(2), 174-178. (5)

*Olney, P.N., & Olney, R.S. (1993). Harlequin ichthyosis among the Navajo: Counseling issues. *Journal of Genetic Counseling, 2*(1), 3-8. (6)

*Strauss, R.P. (1988). Genetic counseling in the cross cultural context: The case of highly observant Judaism. *Patient Education and Counseling, 11*, 43-52. (10)

*Wang, V., & Marsh, F.H. (1992). Ethical principles and cultural integrity in health care delivery: Asian ethnocultural perspectives in genetic services. *Journal of Genetic Counseling, 1*(1), 81-92. (12)

Web Sites

Healthweb Genetics, http://www.lib.umich.edu/libhome/hw/genetics.html This page is maintained by the University of Michigan; it lists other resources at http://www.sph.umich.edu/genetics/phgweb.htm; it also provides information about a student organization, the Public Health Genetics Society, devoted to promoting awareness of the relationship between public health and genetics.

Human Genome Project Information, http://www.ornl.gov/TechResource/Human_Genome/home.html

Primer on Molecular Genetics, http://www.gdb.org/Dan/DOE/intro.html This primer was prepared by Denise Casey (Human Genome Management Information System—Oak Ridge National Laboratory) for the 1991-92 DOE Human Genome Program Report and modified for Web access by the Department of Energy (DOE); 44 pages in Adobe Acrobat format

"A Question of Genes: Inherited Risks" (PBS special, aired Sept. 16, 1997). Noel Schwerin and Graham Chedd, producers. For more information go to http://www.pbs.org/gene/welcome/1_welcome.html

Session 4—Health Behavior / Stress and Illness
Total readings: 60 pages

*Dula, A. (1994). African American suspicion of the health care system is justified: What do we do about it? *Cambridge Quarterly of Health Care Ethics, 3*, 347-357. (11)

Jackson, L.E. (1993). Understanding, eliciting and negotiating clients' multicultural health beliefs. *Nurse Practitioner, 18*(4), 30, 32, 37-38. (4)

*Lerman, C., & Glanz, K. (1997). Stress, coping, and health behavior. In K. Glanz, F.M. Lewis, & B. Rimer (Eds.), *Health behavior and health education: Theory, research, and practice* (2nd ed., pp. 113-138). San Francisco: Jossey-Bass. (26)

*Strecher, V.J., & Rosenstock, I.M. (1997). The health belief model. In K. Glanz, F.M. Lewis, & B.K. Rimer (Eds.), *Health behavior and health education: Theory, research, and practice,* (2nd ed., pp. 41-59). San Francisco: Jossey-Bass. (19)

Session 5—Family Systems, Illness and Disability
Total Readings: 39 pages

*Boss, P. (1988). Definitions: A guide to family stress theory. In *Family stress management.* Newbury Park: Sage. (26)

*Rolland, J.S. (1994). Overview of family dynamics with chronic disorders. In *Families, illness, & disability* (pp. 63-75). New York: Basic Books. (13)

Session 6—Prenatal Development & Infancy
Total Readings: 28 pages + 1 article
  Gottwald, S., & Thurman, S. (1990). Parent–infant interaction in neonatal intensive care units: Implications for research and service delivery. *Infants and Young Children*, 2(3), 1-9. (9)

  *Turner, R. (1995). Black–white infant mortality differential has grown in recent decades and will persist into next century. *Family Planning Perspectives*, 27(6), 267-268. (2) [available online at http://www.jstor.org/fcgi-bin/jstor/viewitem.fcg/00147354/di975949/97p09602/0?config=jstor&frame=frame&userID=980227b1@unc.edu%2f8dd402c9005094283&dpi=3]

  Wheeler, S.F. (1993). Substance abuse during pregnancy. *Primary Care*, 1, 191-207. (17)

Read one article from the following selection:
  *Boone, M. (1989). History, demography, and inner-city Black health. In *Capital crime: Black infant mortality in America* (pp. 53-84). Beverly Hills, CA: Sage. (32)

  *Scott, M.D., & Stern, P.N. (1986). The ethno-market theory: Factors influencing childbearing health practices of northern Louisiana Black women. In P.N. Stern (Ed.), *Women, health, and culture* (pp. 45-60). Washington, DC: Hemisphere. (16)

  *Balcazar, H., & Aoyama, C. (1991). Interpretative views on Hispanic's perinatal problems of low birth weight and prenatal care. *Public Health Reports*, 106(4), 421-426. (6)

  *Krajewski-Jaime, E.R. (1991). Folk-healing among Mexican-American families as a consideration in the delivery of child welfare and child health care services. *Child Welfare*, 70(2), 157-167. (11)

  *Queiro-Tajalli, I. (1989). Hispanic women's perceptions and use of prenatal health care services. *Affilia*, 4(2), 60-72. (13)

Web Sites
  Child Health Research Project (CHR), http://ihl.sph.jhu.edu/chr/chr.htm This project is a collaboration between the World Health Organization (WHO), Harvard University, the ICDDR, Center for Health and Population Research, and the Johns Hopkins Institute, and is devoted to researching ways to improve the management of several common illnesses that affect children.

  CDC Infants' and Children's Health Page, http://www.cdc.gov/diseases/infant.html

  March of Dimes Birth Defects Foundation, http://www.modimes.org

  Maternal and Child Health Bureau, http://www.os.dhhs.gov/hrsa/mchb

  Maternal and Infant Health, http://www.cdc.gov/nccdphp/m_infant.htm

  National Center for Education in Maternal and Child Health, http://www.ncemch.org/

Session 7—Preschool & School Age Years; Interview Assignment due
Total Readings: approx. 82 pages
  *Bibace, R., & Walsh, M.E. (1979). Developmental stages in children's conceptions of illness. In G.C. Stone, F. Cohen, & N.E. Adler (Eds.), *Health psychology—A handbook* (pp. 285-301). Washington, DC: Jossey-Bass. (16)

  *Chesler, M.A., Allswede, J., & Barbarin, O. (1991). Voices from the margin of the family: Siblings of children with cancer. *Journal of Psychosocial Oncology*, 9(4), 19-42. (24)

  Garland, C.W. (1993). Beyond chronic sorrow: A new understanding of family adaptation. In A.P. Turnbull, et al. (Eds.), *Cognitive coping, families, & disability*, (pp. 67-80). Baltimore, MD: Paul H. Brookes. (14)

*Groce, N.E., & Zola, I.K. (1993). Multiculturalism, chronic illness and disability. *Pediatrics*, *91*(5), 1048-1055. (8)

*Meyer, D.J. (Ed.). (1995). *Uncommon fathers: Reflections on raising a child with a disability*. Bethesda, MD: Woodbine House. (Book is in the 5th floor Resource Room—read at least one chapter.)

Web Sites

Bright Futures, http://www.brightfutures.org/index.html

Center for Child Health and Mental Health Policy, http://www.dml.georgetown.edu/depts/ pediatrics/gucdc/policy1.html

Center for the Future of Children, The David and Lucille Packard Foundation, http:// www.futureofchildren.org

Child Health Research Project, http://ih1.sph.jhu.edu/chr/chr.htm

National Center for Children in Poverty, http://cpmcnet.columbia.edu/dept/nccp/

National Information Center for Children and Youth with Disabilities (NICYD/NICHCY), http:// www.nichcy.org

National Institute of Child Health and Human Development, http://wwww.nih.gov/nichd

National Parent Network on Disabilities (NPND), http://www.npnd.org/

Trends in the Well-being of America's Children and Youth 1997 Edition, http://aspe.os.dhhs.gov/ hsp/97trends/intro-web.htm

Zero to Three: www.zerotothree.org

Session 8—Adolescence
Total Readings: 69 pages

Howard, D.E. (1996). Searching for resilience among African American youth exposed to community violence: Theoretical issues. *Journal of Adolescent Health*, *18*(4), 254-262. (9)

*Jessor, R. (1992). Risk behavior in adolescence: A psychosocial framework for understanding and action. In D. Rogers & E. Ginzberg (Eds.), *Adolescents at risk: Medical and social perspectives* (pp. 19-34). Boulder, CO: Westview. (16)

*Rounds, K.A. (1997). Preventing sexually transmitted infections among adolescents. In M.W. Fraser (Ed.), *Risk and resilience in childhood* (pp. 171-194). Washington, DC: NASW Press. (24)

Sells, C.W., & Blum, R.W. (1996). Morbidity and mortality among U.S. adolescents: An overview of data and trends. *American Journal of Public Health*, *86*(4), 513-519. (7)

Smith, C.A. (1997). Factors associated with early sexual activity among urban adolescents. *Social Work*, *42*(4), 334-46. (13)

Web Sites

American Social Health Association, http://sunsite.unc.edu/ASHA/

National Center for Injury Prevention and Control, http://www.cdc.gov/ncipc/dvp/yvfacts.htm

National Center for Youth with Disabilities, http://www.cyfc.umn.edu/Youth/ncyd.html

Sexuality Information and Education Council of the U.S. (SIECUS), http://www.siecus.org/

SIECUS Adolescent Sexuality Bibliography, http://www.siecus.org/pubs/biblio/bibs0001.html
SIECUS has some excellent bibliography pages; several are included here.

YouthInfo, http://youth.os.dhhs.gov/

Session 9—Student Presentations

Session 10—Young Adulthood
Total Readings: 86 pages
  *Gill, C.J. (1996). Becoming visible: Personal health experiences of women with disabilities. In D.M. Krotoski, M.A. Nosek, & M.A. Turk (Eds.), *Women with disabilities: Achieving and maintaining health and well-being* (pp. 5-15). Baltimore, MD: Paul H. Brookes. (10)

  *Schover, L.R., & Jensen, B.J. (1988). "Sexuality and chronic illness: An integrative model" and " Emotional factors and sexuality in chronic illness." In *Sexuality and chronic illness* (pp. 3-13 and 62-77). New York: Guilford. (27) [peruse]

  *Stevens, P.E. (1994). Protective strategies of lesbian clients in health care environments. *Research in Nursing and Health, 17,* 217-229. (13)

  *Zierler, S., & Krieger, N. (1997). Reframing women's risk: Social inequalities and HIV infection. *Annual Review of Public Health, 18,* 401-436. (36)

Web Sites
CDC National Aids Clearinghouse, http://www.cdcnac.org/

HIV Insite, http://hivinsite.ucsf.edu/

SIECUS Sexuality and Disability Bibliography, http://www.siecus.org/pubs/biblio/bibs0011.html

Session 11—Student Presentations

Session 12—Middle Adult Years
Total Readings: 62 pages + perusal (Rodin)
  Biegel, D.E., Sales, E., & Schulz, R. (1991). Caregiving in heart disease (Chp. 4). In *Family caregiving in chronic illness* (pp. 105-128). Newbury Park, CA: Sage. (24)

  *Bricker-Jenkins, M. (1994). Feminist practice and breast cancer: "The patriarchy has claimed my right breast..." *Social Work in Health Care, 19*(3/4), 17-42. (26)

  *Mathews, H.F., Lannin, D.R., & Mitchell, J.P. (1994). Coming to terms with advanced breast cancer: Black women's narratives from eastern North Carolina. *Social Science and Medicine, 38*(6), 789-800. (12)

  *Rodin, G., Craven, J., & Littlefield, C. (1991). "Psychological factors" and "Social factors." In *Depression in the medically ill: An integrated approach* (pp. 3-70 and 181-213). New York: Brunner/ Mazel. (101) [peruse]

Web Sites
American Cancer Society, http://www.cancer.org/frames.html

American Heart Association, http://www.amhrt.org/

American Women's Health Association (AWHA) Health Topics, http://www.amwa-doc.org/healthtopics/healthlist.html

Heart Information Network, http://www.heartinfo.org/

National Cancer Institute, http://www.nci.nih.gov/

SIECUS Sexuality in Middle and Later Life Bibliography, http://www.siecus.org/pubs/biblio/
bibs0014.html

Women's Health Initiative (WHI), http://www.nhlbi.nih.gov/nhlbi/whi1/

Y-Me National Breast Cancer Organization, http://www.y-me.org/

Session 13 Student Presentations

Session 14 Older Adulthood
Total Readings: 110 pages

Cwikel, J., & Fried, A.V. (1992). The social epidemiology of falls among community-dwelling elderly:
Guidelines for prevention. *Disability and Rehabilitation, 14*(3), 113-121. (9)

*Hume, A.L., & Owens, N.J. (1995). Drugs and the elderly. In Reichel (Ed.), *Care of the elderly patient:
Evaluation, diagnosis, and management* (pp. 41-63). Baltimore, MD: Williams and Wilkins. (23)

*National Institute on Aging. (1995). Alzheimer's Disease: Unraveling the mystery. NIH Publication
No. 95-3782, Bethesda, MD. (48)

Pearlin, L., Mullan, J.T., Semple, S.J., Skaff, M.M. (1990). Caregiving and the stress process: An
overview of concepts and their measures. *The Gerontologist, 30*(5), 583-594. (12)

*Reynolds, C.F. (1995). Recognition and differentiation of elderly depression in the clinical setting.
Geriatrics, 50(SUPP1), S6-S15. (10)

Wilson-Ford, V. (1992). Health-protective behaviors of rural black elderly women. *Health and Social
Work, 17*(1), 28-36. (9)

Web Sites

Alzheimer's Disease Education and Referral (ADEAR) Center, http://www.alzheimers.org/

Health Net—Senior's Health, http://www.health-net.com/seniors.htm

Healthtouch Online—Older Americans, http://www.healthtouch.com/level1/leaflets/102179/
102179.htm

National Institute of Neurological Disorders and Stroke (NINDS), http://www.ninds.nih.gov/

National Institute on Aging, http://www.nih.gov/nia/

Osteoporosis and Related Bone Diseases—National Resource Center (ORBD-NRC), http://
www.osteo.org/

Session 15—Older Adulthood; Distribute Final Exam

Session 16—Death and Bereavement
Total Readings: 89 pages

*McNeil, J.S. (1995). Bereavement and loss. In R.L. Edwards (Ed.-in-Chief), *Encyclopedia of social work*
(19th ed., pp. 284-291). Washington, DC: NASW Press. (8)

*Rando, T.A. (1986). *Grief, dying and death: Clinical interventions for caregivers* (pp. 199-250).
Champaign, IL: Research Press. (52)

*Shapiro, E.R. (1996). Family bereavement and cultural diversity: A social development perspec-
tive. *Family Process, 35*(3), 313-332. (20)

Wortman, C.B., & Silver, R.C. (1989). The myths of coping with loss. *Journal of Consulting and Clinical Psychology, 57*(3), 349-357. (9)

Web Sites

Bereavement Education Center, http://www.bereavement.org/

Growth House, Inc., http://www.growthhouse.org/default.html Growth House calls their organization the "international gateway to resources for life-threatening illness and end of life issues"; very comprehensive site.

SUPPLEMENTAL READINGS

Aday, L.A. (1993). *At risk in America.* San Francisco: Jossey Bass.

Barth, J.C. (1993). *It runs in my family: Overcoming the legacy of family illness.* New York: Brunner/ Mazel.

Blackman, J.A. (1990). *Medical aspects of developmental disabilities in children birth to three.* (2nd ed.) The Division of Developmental Disabilities, Dept. of Pediatrics, University of Iowa.

Braithwaite, R.L., & Taylor, S.E. (Eds.). (1992). *Health issues in the Black community.* San Francisco: Jossey-Bass.

Charmaz, K. (1991). *Good days, bad days: The self in chronic illness and time.* New Brunswick, NJ: Rutgers University Press.

Chilman, C.S., Nunnally, E.W., & Cox, F.M. (Eds.). (1988). *Chronic illness and disability.* Beverly Hills, CA: Sage.

Corbin, J., & Strauss, A. (1988). *Unending work and care: Managing chronic illness.* San Francisco: Jossey-Bass.

Hobbs, N., Perrin, J.M., & Ireys, H.T. (1985). *Chronically ill children and their families.* San Francisco: Jossey-Bass.

Hockenberry, J. (1995). *Moving violations.* New York: Hyperion.

Hymovich, D.P., & Hagopian, G.A. (1992). *Chronic illness in children and adults: A psychosocial approach.* Philadelphia: Saunders.

Healthy people 2000: Midcourse review and 1995 revisions. (1995). Washington, DC: U.S. Department of Health and Human Resources, U.S. Public Health Service.

Healthy people 2000: National health promotion and disease prevention objectives: Full report with commentary. (1991). (U.S. Department of Health and Human Services Publication No. PHS 91-50212). Washington, DC: U.S. Government Printing Office.

Irwin, C.E., Brindis, C.D., Brodt, S.E., Bennett, T.A., & Rodrigues, R.Q. (1991). *The health of America's youth: Current trends in health status and utilization of health services.* San Francisco: University of California at San Francisco.

Isaacs, M.R. (1992). *Violence: The impact of community violence on African American children and families.* Arlington, VA: National Center for Education in Maternal and Child Health.

Nuland, S.B. (1994). *How we die: Reflections on life's final chapter.* New York: Knopf.

Pollin, I. (1994). *Taking charge: Overcoming the challenge of long-term illness.* New York: Random House.

Register, C. (1987). *Living with chronic illness.* New York: Free Press.

Rodin, G., Craven, J., & Littlefield, C. (1991). *Depression in the medically ill.* New York: Brunner/Mazel.

Rogers, D., & Ginzberg, E. (Eds.). (1992). *Adolescents at risk: Medical and social perspectives.* Boulder, CO: Westview.

Rosen, E.J. (1990). *Families facing death.* Lexington, MA: Lexington Books.

Schwartz, A., & Schwartz, R.M. (1993). *Depression: Theories and treatments.* New York: Columbia University Press.

Seligman, M., & Darling, R.B. (1989). *Ordinary families, special children: A systems approach to childhood disability.* New York: Guilford.

Stroebe, W., & Stroebe, M.S. (1987). *Bereavement and health: The psychological and physical consequences of partner loss.* New York: Cambridge University Press.

Wallace, H.M., Nelson, R.P., & Sweeney, P.J. (Eds.). (1994). *Maternal and child health practice* (4th ed.). Oakland, CA: Third Party.

Worden, J.W. (1991). *Grief counseling and grief therapy: A handbook for the mental health practitioner.* New York: Springer.

Worden, J.W. (1996). *Children and grief: When a parent dies.* New York: Guilford.

APPENDIX

Final Exam

This exam is due by 5:00 p.m. on Monday, December 7, 1998. All exams should be typed, double-spaced, and *edited*. Your response to each question should be between three and four pages. *It is important that you cite readings to support your responses.* Cite all references using APA style, for example (Gill, 1996). This is an open book exam; you may use any *non-human sources* to prepare your answers. Observe the Honor Code and do not discuss the contents of this exam with anyone. You will be graded on how well you: (1) integrate course readings, lecture material, and class discussions; (2) conceptualize and critically analyze information; and (3) follow directions as specified for each question.

Put your Personal Identification Number on the exam. Do not put your name on the exam.

I. Respond to *one* of the following two questions:

    A. In our readings and discussion regarding the relationship between stress and disease, we covered several models: the Contextual Model of Family Stress (Boss, 1988, p. 28), the "Transactional Model of Stress and Coping" presented in the chapter by Lerman and Glanz (1997, p. 116), and a conceptual model of caregivers' stress (Pearlin, Mullan, Semple, & Skaff, 1990, p. 586). Apply one of these models to a case example of an individual or family confronted with a major illness or threat to health (i.e., walk the reader through the model). In your response identify (1) the stressor, (2) the outcome, and (3) key variables that influence the relationship between the stressor and the outcome. Explain how these variables influence the relationship between the stressor and the outcome. *Briefly* describe how you would intervene with this individual or family to reduce the impact of the health-related stressor on the outcome.

    OR

    B. The Health Belief Model (Strecher & Rosenstock, 1997) was originally developed to explain individuals' preventive health behavior; it has also been applied to the explanation of illness and sick-role behavior. Select a specific disease or health problem (one that has been discussed in the readings, presentations, or in class) and use the Health Belief Model to explain preventive, illness, *or* sick-role behavior related to this disease or health problem (i.e., walk the reader thorough the model). Your response should cover each of the major components of the model and how they relate to one another. *Briefly* explain how you would use the Health Belief Model in working with a client who is trying to make a decision about or take action related to the health problem you have described. (The best way to respond to this question is to use a case example).

II. Respond to *one* of the following five questions (A–E).

A. We have focused on the impact of illness, disability, and health problems on individual development and family functioning. Compare and contrast the impact of a disease, disability, or health problem (e.g., cancer, arthritis, HIV infection, Alzheimer's disease, etc.) on individual and family development and functioning if it were to occur at two different life stages. For example, how would the experience of developing leukemia in adolescence be different than in the middle years? In your response discuss effects on identity, family and peer relationships, educational or vocational status, financial resources, sexuality, and biopsychosocial development. How does the individual's developmental stage influence his/her ability to understand and cope with this illness, disability, or health problem? When responding to this question, select an illness, disability, or health problem other than the one you used for question I. In addition to other readings, use the Rolland chapter to respond to this question.

OR

B. In the class session on the epidemiology of health and disease, we discussed factors that are related to mortality and morbidity. Discuss how each of these factors affect infant mortality. Include in your discussion an explanation of how these factors may interact resulting in higher infant mortality.

OR

C. A major cause of mortality and morbidity in adolescence is engagement in risky behavior. Apply one of the models or conceptual frameworks *covered in the course session on adolescence* to explain why adolescents might engage in a particular risky behavior (e.g., substance use, unprotected or early sexual activity, violence, driving while intoxicated). Briefly critique the model or conceptual framework that you have chosen in terms of usefulness and fit. In your response address incidence/prevalence, causes (known or hypothesized), and possible interventions.

OR

D. Choose *two* of the following vignettes to discuss the bio-psychosocial impact of grief and bereavement on individuals, families, and communities. Include (a) the factors that influence bereavement adaptation; and (b) the psychological and social impact of the loss on the survivors (e.g., how might survivors in vignette "1" adjust as compared to survivors in vignette "3").

1. An 82-year-old African-American woman dies at home of breast cancer surrounded by family and friends after a prolonged, debilitating period of treatment. She is survived by her husband of 63 years, three children, nine grandchildren, and seven great grandchildren. This large extended family has lived in a rural community in eastern North Carolina for generations.

2. A 41-year-old white married woman who is in recovery (from alcoholism) with two adolescent boys discovers her husband's suicide note after finding him slumped over the steering wheel of his truck. Their 20-year marriage had been particularly difficult during the previous 5 years.

3. A 5-week-old Hispanic male infant dies in the neonatal intensive care unit at UNC Hospitals. He was born at 24 weeks gestation with several major birth anomalies; his mother had not received any prenatal care. Both parents live in rural North Carolina, about an hour from the hospital, where they work as migrant laborers during the summer harvest. They came to North Carolina from Mexico eight months ago. The surviving family includes three other children, all girls (ages 12, 5, and 2).

4. A 13-year-old white female commits suicide by shooting herself in the head in a restroom at a local middle school. Several of her friends knew that she had come to school with a gun and had told her that they would talk with the principal if she didn't get rid of the gun. She was an excellent student and well liked by the younger children in her neighborhood for whom she frequently babysat. She is survived by her mother and stepfather.

5. A 12-year-old African-American male dies at UNC Hospitals after a 6-year struggle with leukemia. He is survived by his 14-year-old sister, 9-year-old brother, and both parents. The family lives two hours from the hospital and his mother quit her job a year ago when he had a bone marrow transplant because she had to spend so much time at the hospital. During the last year of his illness, his parents separated and his father moved out of the home.

6. A 55-year-old white gay man dies of AIDS after living with his illness for the past 12 years. He had been estranged from his family (living in a small town in North Carolina) since "coming out" in his late twenties. He and his partner had both been active in the gay community in Charlotte. His partner of 25 years also has AIDS but is doing well since he began a new drug regimen.

OR

E. Mrs. C. is an 87-year-old African-American widow living in a rural North Carolina community. Since her husband of 60 years died 7 years ago from a stroke, she has lived alone. Prior to his death, Mrs. C. cared for her husband; he was disabled for several years from an earlier stroke and also was suffering from complications of adult onset diabetes. Since her husband's death, she has been able to function relatively well with the assistance of a weekly homemaker/chore worker. She has continued to be active in her church, and various members have provided transportation so that she could attend services and other church activities. Her son, Mr. J.. and his wife live two hours away. Up until 9 months ago, they visited Mrs. C. almost every weekend. However, during the past year, Mr. J. had a massive heart attack and his wife, Mrs. J., who is also in poor health due to her uncontrolled diabetes, have not been able to visit very often. During the last year, Mrs. C.'s functional status has been deteriorating. She has been falling twice a week on average, her systolic hypertension has not been controlled, she has become increasingly forgetful and confused. Mrs. C.'s Department of Social Services social worker reports that Mrs. C. "just doesn't seem to have the energy that she used to have" and wonders how much longer she can continue to live on her own. The social worker wants Mrs. C. to see her family doctor whom she hasn't seen for 14 months. However, Mrs. C. is reluctant to do so; she prefers to treat her aches and pains with over-the-counter medicines—although she occasionally takes some of the medications that were prescribed by her doctor over a year ago. In addition, she feels that her doctor will not be able to do anything more for her.

1. How representative is Mrs. C. of others in her age group?

2. What are some of the possible causes of her falling so frequently?

3. What problems might she be encountering with her medication regimen?

4. Given the limited information you have about Mrs. C. and what you know about other people of her age, what major health problems is she at risk for developing? If she should develop these problems, what might be the most likely outcome and why?

5. What are some of the constraints and facilitators for Mrs. C. in managing her current condition?

University of Chicago
School of Social Service Administration and
Harris Graduate School of Public Policy Studies
Chicago, IL

Course Title: Clinical Social Work Issues in Health Care (SSA 407, 519; PubPol 368)
Fall 1996

Course Instructor: Sarah Gehlert

DOMAIN AND BOUNDARIES

This course introduces students to some of the issues and tasks facing social workers and other professionals in a variety of health care settings. These include working on teams, on interprofessional teams, recognizing cultural biases in medicine and how they affect social work practice, and understanding the determinants of health behavior. Value and ethical conflicts inherent in clinical practice in health care are emphasized, with special attention to issues related to women, minorities, the aged, and the poor.

OBJECTIVES

A. To acquire an understanding of the role of clinical issues in diverse health care settings.

B. To develop an understanding of what it means to be a member of an interdisciplinary health care team and what factors influence team functioning.

C. To understand and use basic medical terminology.

D. To acquire an understanding of the problems inherent in communication between health care professionals and patients and families, with emphasis on situations in which the two groups have different cultural constructions of reality. An understanding of the link between health care communication and outcomes should also be acquired.

E. To be able to articulate the importance of eliciting personal and group health belief models for positive health care outcomes.

F. To gain an understanding of the complexities inherent in the application and use of clinical interventions in different health care settings and systems of health care delivery.

G. To recognize how an understanding of theories of health behavior can be used to enhance clinical effectiveness.

TEXTS

Required

Sontag, S. (1978). *Illness as metaphor.* New York: Farrar, Strauss and Giroux.

Course packet. The course packet contains all required readings. It can be purchased in the SSA production room. Optional readings are on reserve in the SSA library.

Optional

Balshem, M. (1993). *Cancer in the community*. Washington, DC: Smithsonian Institution Press.

Chabner, D. (1991). *Medical terminology: A short course*. Philadelphia: W.B. Saunders.

Glanz, K., Lewis, F.M., & Rimer, B.K. (Eds.). (1990). *Health behavior and health education: Theory, research, and practice*. San Francisco: Jossey-Bass.

Snow, L.F. (1993). *Walkin' over medicine*. Boulder, CO: Westview.

ORGANIZATION

The class meets for three hours per week. Attendance is required at all sessions. The format of the course includes lecture and class discussion. Readings are to be completed prior to the session for which they are assigned. Readings appear on the syllabus in the order in which they will be discussed in class.

GRADING CRITERIA

Performance will be evaluated on two written assignments and class participation. Weightings toward the final course grade are as follows:

Assignment #1......................40%

Assignment #2......................40%

Participation..........................20%

Written assignments which are turned in after their due dates will be lowered by one-half letter grade.

Students must inform the instructor by the end of the fourth week of if they wish to have their performance graded Pass/D/Fail.

ASSIGNMENT DETAILS

Assignment #1

The purpose of this assignment is to apply the theories of health behavior discussed in class to a specific health issue or problem. Students should choose one of the articles or sets of articles offered ("Second Wave of AIDS Feared by Officials in San Francisco" and "Flirting with Suicide" or "Yeh, I'm Trying to Quit"). They should then select two theories which they think allow an understanding of the health behavior described in the article. Next, they should analyze the health behavior in terms of each of the two theories. Lastly, students should make a strong case for which of the two theories best accounts for why the health behavior is as it is (e.g., why teens ignore health warnings about smoking).

The paper should include a brief outline of the theory and of the issue (written succinctly, but providing sufficient information to assess an individual student's level of understanding of each). Next, it should provide a detailed analysis of how the theory fits the situation described. Are all of the salient elements of the situation described covered by the theory? Is the theory adequate to explain the behavior? Does the theory allow for a better understanding of the behavior discussed in the article than would an atheoretical analysis? If not, why not? This should be the meat of the paper. Lastly, the implications for practice of using this theory to try to understand the behavior described in the two articles should be addressed. Lastly, the student should make a choice as to which of the two theories best explains the behavior in question and why.

The final product will be due at the beginning of Session 4. It should not exceed 10 pages in length.

Assignment #2

Students may choose *one* of the following two assignments:

Choice #1—Interview a clinician in the community who treats patients using nontraditional health care practices, such as homeopathy, acupuncture, herbalism, *espiritismo*, or *curanderismo*. The following information should be obtained and included in the paper: (1) the history of use over time of the nontraditional health care technique, emphasizing its cultural origins, if applicable; (2) specifically how the technique works; (3) indications for its use; (4) contraindications for its use; (4) your reaction to its effectiveness.

Choice #2—This can be a small-group activity (2–4 persons). Following Balshem's lead in "Project CAN-DO," interview five individuals of the same culture group (per person, all from either the same or different culture groups [the latter is obviously more complex]; culture group is here defined as people sharing the same health belief system) to determine their conception of two health conditions of your choosing (Balshem used cancer and heart disease). Make your choice meaningful, i.e., choose two conditions that you expect to differ, based on what you have learned in the course. Questions should include but not be limited to: (1) "What comes to mind when you think about (each of the two conditions) the disease itself?"; (2) "Can you explain your own idea of what goes on inside the body with (each of the two conditions)?"; and, (3) "How would you explain this to someone 12 years old?" Add whatever other questions you think would allow you an understanding of how respondents view the two conditions and how their conceptions fit into other aspects of their social systems. How do their conceptions differ from that of the medical community, if at all? Pull the information together into a conceptual scheme like those of Sontag or Balshem. How does this information help you better understand the group and provide guidance for planning health education efforts?

Assignment 2 is due at Session 10. The written assignment should not exceed 15 pages in length. Each individual (Choice 1) or group (Choice 2) should be prepared to present in class.

SCHEDULE

Session 1
Overview of the course
History of concern with clinical issues in health care
The present state of clinical concerns in health care

Required Reading

Noble, H.B. (1995, July 3). Quality is focus of health plans. *New York Times*, pp. 1, 16.

Staff. (1995, August 27). Medicaid cuts may leave more people uninsured. *Chicago Tribune*, p. 4.

Mahowald, M.B. (1993). *Women and children in health care: An unequal majority.* New York: Oxford University Press. Chapter 2, "Sex-roles and stereotypes in health care"

Carroll, D., Smith, G.D., & Bennett, P. (1996). Some observations on health and socioeconomic status. *Journal of Health Psychology, 1,* 23-39.

Berkman, B., Bonander, E., Rutchick, I., Silverman, I., Kemler, B., Marcus, L., & Isaacson-Rubinosa, M-J. (1990). Social work in health care: Directions in practice. *Social Science and Medicine, 31,* 19-26.

Optional Reading

Holosko, M. (1989). Social work practice roles in health care: Daring to be different. In M.J. Holosko & P.A. Taylor (Eds.), *Social work practice in health care settings* (pp. 21-31). Toronto: Canadian Scholars' Press.

Nacman, M. (1980). Social work in health settings: A historical review. In K.W. Davidson & S.S. Clarke (Eds.), *Social work in health care* (pp. 7-22). Binghamton, NY: Haworth.

Taylor, P.A. (1989). New wave social work: Practice roles for the 1990s and beyond. In M.J. Holosko & P.A. Taylor (Eds.), *Social work practice in health care settings* (pp. 639-646). Toronto: Canadian Scholars' Press.

Reynolds, M.M. (1990). The role of social workers in medical education: A historical perspective. In K.W. Davidson & S.S. Clarke (Eds.), *Social work in health care* (pp. 23-37). Binghamton, NY: Haworth.

Lane, H.J. (1982). Toward the preparation of social work specialists in health care. *Health and Social Work, 7,* 230-234.

Sessions 2 and 3
Theories of health behavior:
The Health Beliefs Model
Theory of Reasoned Action
Attribution Theory

Required Reading

Ewart, C.K. (1991). Social action theory for a public health psychology. *American Psychologist, 46,* 931-946.

Rolland, J.S. (1990). The impact of illness on the family. In K.E. Rakel (Ed.), *Textbook of family medicine* (pp. 80-100). Philadelphia: W.B. Saunders.

Optional Reading

Glanz, K., Lewis, F.M., & Rimer, B.K. (Eds.). (1990). *Health behavior and health education: Theory, research, and practice.* San Francisco: Jossey-Bass. Chapters 3–5, "The health belief model: Explaining health behavior through expectancies"; "Health behavior as a rational process: Theory of reasoned action and multiattribute utility theory"; "How causal explanations influence health behavior: Attribution theory".

Session 4
Working on interprofessional teams
Medical communication:
Provider-patient interactions II

Required Reading

Nason, F. (1990). Diagnosing the hospital team. In K.W. Davidson & S.S. Clarke (Eds.), *Social work in health care* (pp. 309-333). Binghamton, NY: Haworth.

Kane, R.A. (1990). The interprofessional team as a small group. In K.W. Davidson & S.S. Clarke (Eds.), *Social work in health care* (pp. 277-294). Binghamton, NY: Haworth.

Mailick, M.D., & Jordan, P. (1990). A multimodal approach to collaborative practice in health setting. In K.W. Davidson & S.S. Clarke (Eds.), *Social work in health care* (pp. 295-307). Binghamton, NY: Haworth.

Northouse, P.G., & Northouse, L.L. (1985). *Health communication: A handbook for health professionals.* Englewood Cliffs, NJ: Prentice Hall. Chapter 6, "Small group communication in health care."

Roberts, C. (1989). Conflicting professional values in social work and medicine. *Health and Social Work*, 14, 211-218.

Joos, S.K., & Hickam, D.H. (1990). How health professionals influence health behavior: Patient-provider interaction and health care. In K. Glanz, F.M. Lewis, & B.K. Rimer (Eds.), *Health behavior and health education* (pp. 216-241). San Francisco: Jossey-Bass.

Session 5
Medical communication:
Provider-patient interactions II
Terminology
Abbreviations

Required Reading

Beckman, H.B., & Frankel, R.M. (1984). The effect of physician behavior on the collection of data. *Annals of Internal Medicine, 101*, 692-696.

Greenfield, S., Kaplan, S., & Ware, J.E. (1985). Expanding patient involvement in care. *Annals of Internal Medicine, 102*, 520-528.

Kaplan, S.H., Greenfield, S., & Ware, J.E. (1989). Assessing the effects of physician-patient interactions on the outcomes of chronic disease. *Medical Care, 27*, S110-S127.

Samora, J., Saunders, L., & Larson, R.F. (1969). Medical vocabulary knowledge among hospital patients. *Journal of Health and Human Behavior, 22*, 83-92.

Slomski, A.J. (1993, May 24). Making sure that your care doesn't get lost in the translation. *Medical Economics*, pp. 122-139.

Sideris, D.A., Tsouna-Hadjis, S.T., Toumanidis, P.E., Vardas, P.E., & Moulopoulos, S.D. (1986). Attitudinal educational objectives at therapeutic consultation: Measures of performance, educational approach and evaluation. *Medical Education, 20*, 307-313.

Optional Reading

Brown, J.B., Weston, W.W., Stewart, M., McCracken, E.C., & McWhinney, I. (1989). Patient-centered clinical interviewing. In M. Stewart & D. Roter (Eds.), *Communicating with medical patients* (pp. 107-120). Newbury Park, CA: Sage.

Scott, N., & Weiner, M.F. (1984). "Patientspeak": An exercise in communication. *Journal of Medical Education, 59*, 890-893.

Session 6
Belief systems

Required Reading

Sontag, S. (1978). *Illness as metaphor.* New York: Farrar, Strauss and Giroux.

Balshem, M. (1993). *Cancer in the community.* Washington, DC: Smithsonian Institution Press. Chapter 3, "Project CAN-DO."

Snow, L.F. (1993). *Walkin' over medicine.* Boulder, CO: Westview. Chapters 2, 6, 8, & 9 in course packet. Note: Each student will be assigned one of the four chapters.

Optional Reading

Kirmayer. L.J. (1992). The body's insistence on meaning: Metaphor as presentation and representation in illness experience. *Medical Anthropology Quarterly, 6,* 323-346.

Sontag, S. (1989). *AIDS and its metaphors.* New York: Farrar, Strauss and Giroux.

Weston, W.W., & Brown, J.B. (1989). The importance of patients' beliefs. In M. Stewart & D. Roter (Eds.), *Communicating with medical patients* (pp. 77-85). Newbury Park, CA: Sage.

Session 7
Cognitive factors in health and illness
Personality and health
Stress and coping

Required Reading

Taylor, S., & Brown, J.D. (1988). Illusion and well-being: A social psychological perspectiveo n mental health. *Psychological Bulletin, 103,* 193-210.

Taylor, S.E. (1983). Adjustment to threatening events: A theory of cognitive adaptation. *American Psychologist,* 1161-1173.

Taylor, S. (1992). Optimism, coping, psychological distress, and high-risk sexual behavior among men at risk for acquired immunodeficiency syndrome (AIDS). *Journal of Personality and Social Psychology, 63,* 460-473.

Session 9
Cultural factors in health care practice
Alternative belief systems

Required Reading

Pachter, L.M. (1994). Culture and clinical care: Folk illness beliefs and behaviors and their implications for health care delivery. *Journal of the American Medical Association, 271,* 690-694.

Eisenberg, D.M., Kessler, R.C., Foster, C., Norlock, F.E., Calkins, D.R., & Delbanco, T.L. (1993). Unconventional medicine in the United States. *New England Journal of Medicine, 328,* 246-252.

Kleinman, A., Eisenberg, L., & Good, B. (1978). Culture, illness, and care: Clinical lessons from anthropologic and cross-cultural research. *Annals of Internal Medicine, 88,* 251-258.

Brownlee, A. (1978). The family and health care: Explorations in cross-cultural settings. *Social Work and Health Care, 4,* 179-198.

Low, S.M. (1984). The cultural basis of health, illness and disease. *Social Work in Health Care, 9,* 13-23.

Optional Reading

D'Andrade, R.G. (1973). Cultural constructions of reality. In L. Nader & T.W. Maretzki (Eds.), *Cultural illness and health* (pp. 115-127). Washington, DC: American Anthropological Association.

Dalton, H. (1991). AIDS in blackface. In N.F. McKenzie (Ed.), *The AIDS reader: Social, political, ethical issues* (pp. 122-139). New York: Meridian.

Turner, F.J. (1990). Social work practice theory: A trans-cultural resource for health care. *Social Science and Medicine, 31,* 13-17.

Sessions 9 and 10
Clinical interventions in health care:
Beyond the medical model
Overview
Assessing psychiatric problems

Required Reading

Coulton, C.J. (1981). Person-environment fit as the focus in health care. *Social Work, 26*, 26-34.

Nacman, M. (1990). A systems approach to the provision of social work services in health settings. In K.W. Davidson & S.S. Clarke (Eds.), *Social work in health care* (pp. 375-383). Binghamton, NY: Haworth.

Schukit, M.A. (1983). Anxiety related to medical disease. *Journal of Clinical Psychology, 44*, 31-36.

Weick, A. (1983). Issues in overturning a medical model of social work practice. *Social Work, 28*, 467-471.

Optional Reading

Backman, M.E. (1989). *The psychology of the physically ill patient: A clinician's guide.* New York: Plenum Press. Chapter 8, "Suicide"

Rosen, A., Proctor, E.K., & Livne, S. (1985). Planning and direct practice. *Social Service Review, 59*, 161-177.

University of Chicago
School of Social Service Administration and
Department of Health Studies
Chicago, IL

Course Title: Introduction to Health Services Research (HS351/SSA463)
Fall Quarter 1998

Course Instructor: Min-Woong Sohn

OBJECTIVES

The purpose of this course is to introduce students to the principles and methods of conducting health services research. This course covers the following methodological aspects of health services research: scientific approach, definition and concept formation, measurement, research design, modes of observation, and inferential methods. We will devote some time to discuss issues involved in measuring cost of health care, quality of care, and competition. The focus of the course is to help students (1) understand the conceptual foundations of the research process, (2) learn methods of carrying out scientific inquiry in a valid and reliable manner, (3) understand and interpret research findings in health services research, and (4) learn how to prepare a research proposal.

TEXTBOOKS

Required

Shi, Leiyu. 1997. *Health Services Research Methods.* Albany, NY: Delmar.

Sudman, Seymour, and Norman M. Bradburn. 1982. *Asking Questions: A Practical Guide to Questionnaire Design.* San Francisco: Jossey-Bass.

Hempel, Carl G. 1966. *Philosophy of Natural Science.* Englewood Cliffs, NJ: Prentice Hall.

Campbell, Donald T., and Julian C. Stanley. 1963. *Experimental and Quasi-Experimental Designs for Research.* Boston: Houghton Mifflin.

McIver, John P., and Edward G. Carmines. 1981. *Unidimensional Scaling.* Beverly Hills, CA: Sage.

Jacob, Herbert. 1984. *Using Published Data: Errors and Remedies.* Newbury Park, CA: Sage.

Recommended

Kaplan, Abraham. 1998. *The Conduct of Inquiry: Methodology for Behavioral Science.* Scranton, PA: Chandler.

Cook, Thomas D., and Donald T. Campbell. 1979. *Quasi-Experimentation.* Boston: Houghton Mifflin.

Carmines, Edward G., and Richard A. Zeller. 1979. *Reliability and Validity Assessment.* Newbury Park, CA: Sage.

REQUIREMENTS

1. Readings with asterisks (*) are suggested; all the others are required. Reading should be finished before class.

2. One 5-page paper. This is an exercise of operationalization. The concept to measure is "case management." Due Session 4.

3. A research proposal on a topic of student's own choice. The proposal should not exceed 15 double-spaced pages in length, including all tables and figures. It must use the PHS398 forms, which will later be made available to students either in WordPerfect or MS Word formats. Due Session 15.

4. Midterm and final examinations. The midterm exam will be on Session 8, and the final during exam week.

EVALUATION

Class participation	10%
5-page paper	10%
Research proposal	30%
Midterm examination	20%
Final examination	30%

SCHEDULE AND READING ASSIGNMENTS

I. INTRODUCTION

1.   Introduction and Overview

Eisenberg, John M. 1998. "Health Services Research in a Market-Oriented Health Care System." *Health Affairs* 17: 98-108.

Luft, Harold S. 1986. "Health Services Research as a Scientific Process: The Metamorphosis of an Empirical Research Project from Grant Proposal to Final Report." *Health Services Research* 21: 563-584.

Brook, Robert H. 1989. "Health Services Research: Is It Good for You and Me?" *Academic Medicine* 64: 124-130.

Finkelstein, Beth, Shirley Llorens, and Duncan Neuhauser. 1996. "Health Services Research Methods: A Survey of Two Journals." *Medical Care* 34: 987-988.

*Torrens, Paul R. 1993. "Historical Evolution and Overview of Health Services in the United States." Pp. 3-28 in Stephen J. Williams and Paul R. Torrens (Eds.), *Introduction to Health Services*. Albany, NY: Delmar.

*Fraser, Irene. 1997. "Introduction: Research on Health Care Organizations and Markets—The Best and Worst of Times." *Health Services Research* 32: 669-678.

II. NATURE OF SCIENTIFIC INQUIRY

2.   The Scientific Approach

Shi. Chapter 1: Scientific Foundations of Health Services Research.

Cook and Campbell. Chapter 1: Causal Inference and the Language of Experimentation.

Kaplan. Chapters 1 and 9: Methodology, Explanation.

3.   Conceptual Foundations of Research

Shi. Chapter 2: Conceptualizing Health Services Research.

*Kaplan. Chapter 2: Concepts.

Hempel. Chapters 6 and 7: Theories and Theoretical Explanation, Concept Formation.

Seeman, Melvin. 1972. "On the Meaning of Alienation." Pp. 25-34 in Paul Lazarsfeld, Ann Pasanella, and Morris Rosenberg (Eds.), *Continuities in the Language of Social Research.* New York: Free Press.

*Williams, David R. 1994. "The Concept of Race in *Health Services Research:* 1966 to 1990." *Health Services Research* 29: 261-274.

*Lamb, Gerri S. 1992. "Conceptual and Methodological Issues in Nurse Case Management Research." *ANS [Advances in Nursing Science]* 15: 16-24.

*Cook, Tom H. 1998. "The Effectiveness of Inpatient Case Management: Fact or Fiction." *Journal of Nursing Administration* 28: 36-46.

*Gorey, Kevin, Donald R. Leslie, Thom Morris, W. Vince Carruthers, Lindsay John, and James Chacko. 1998. "Effectiveness of Case Management with Severely and Persistently Mentally Ill People." *Community Mental Health Journal* 34: 241-250.

4.   Research Process

Shi. Chapters 3, 4, and 10: Groundwork in Health Services Research, Research Review, Design in Health Services Research.

Babbie, Earl. 1995. *The Practice of Social Research,* 7th Edition. Belmont, CA: Wadsworth. Chapter 4: Research Design.

Luft, Harold. 1986. "Health Services Research as a Scientific Process: The Metamorphosis of an Empirical Research Project from Grant Proposal to Final Report." *Health Services Research* 21: 563-584.

III. RESEARCH DESIGN

5.   Measurement, Validity, and Reliability

Carmines and Zeller. Reliability and Validity Assessment.

*Kaplan. Chapter 5: Measurement.

*Cook and Campbell. Chapter 2: Validity.

6.   Experimental Designs

Shi. Chapter 7: Experimental Research.

*Kaplan. Chapter 4: Experiment.

Campbell and Stanley. Pp. 1-6, 13-34.

*Cook and Campbell. Chapter 8: The Conduct of Randomized Experiments.

Newhouse, Joseph P. 1974. "A Design for a Health Insurance Experiment." *Inquiry* 11: 5-27.

*Newhouse, Joseph P. 1991. "Controlled Experimentation as Research Policy." Pp. 161-194 in Eli Ginzberg (Ed.), *Health Services Research: Key to Health Policy.* Cambridge, MA: Harvard University Press.

*Manning, Willard G., Joseph P. Newhouse, Naihua Duan, Emmett B. Keeler, Arleen Leibowitz, and M. Susan Marquis. 1987. "Health Insurance and the Demand for Medical Care: Evidence from a Randomized Experiment." *The American Economic Review* 77: 251-277.

7.   Pre- and Quasi-Experimental Designs

*Cook and Campbell. Chapters 3 and 5: Quasi-Experiments: Nonequivalent Control Group Designs; Quasi-Experiments: Interrupted Time-Series Designs.

Campbell and Stanley. Pp. 6-13, 34-71.

IV. MODES OF OBSERVATION

8.   Secondary Analysis

Shi. Chapter 5: Secondary Analysis.

*Jacob, Herbert. 1984. *Using Published Data: Errors and Remedies.* Newbury Park, CA: Sage.

Iezzoni, Lisa I. 1997. "Assessing Quality Using Administrative Data." *Annals of Internal Medicine* 127: 666-674.

9.   Observational Methods

Shi. Chapter 6: Qualitative Research.

Stake, Robert E. 1998. "Case Studies." Pp. 86-109 in Norman K. Denzin and Yvonna S. Lincoln (Eds.), *Strategies of Qualitative Inquiry.* Thousand Oaks, CA: Sage.

*Miller, William L., and Benjamin F. Crabtree. 1998. "Clinical Research." Pp. 292-314 in Norman K. Denzin and Yvonna S. Lincoln (Eds.), *Strategies of Qualitative Inquiry.* Thousand Oaks, CA: Sage.

Stange, Kurt C., William L. Miller, Benjamin F. Crabtree, Patrick J. O'Connor, and Stephen J. Zyzanski. 1994. "Multimethod Research: Approaches for Integrating Qualitative and Quantitative Methods." *Journal of General Internal Medicine* 9: 278-282.

*Pope, Catherine, and Nick Mays. 1995. "Reaching the parts other methods cannot reach: an introduction to qualitative methods in health and health services research." *British Medical Journal* 311: 42-45.

*Mays, Nick, and Catherine Pope. 1995. "Observational methods in health care settings." *British Medical Journal* 311: 182-184.

*Kitzinger, Jenny. 1995. "Introducing focus groups." *British Medical Journal* 311: 299-302.

10.   Survey Research

Shi. Chapter 8: Survey Research.

Denzin, Norman K. 1978. *The Research Act.* New York: McGraw-Hill. Chapter 4. "The Sociological Interview."

*Asch, David A., Kathryn Jedrziewski, and Nicholas A. Christakis. 1997. "Response Rates to Mail Surveys Published in Medical Journals." *Journal of Clinical Epidemiology* 50: 1129-1136.

*Sudman and Bradburn. Chapters 7-11.

11.   Questionnaire Construction

Sudman and Bradburn. Chapters 1-5.

12.   Index Construction and Scaling Methods

*Babbie, Earl. 1995. *The Practice of Social Research,* 7th Edition. Belmont, CA: Wadsworth. Chapter 7: Indexes, Scales, and Typologies.

McIver and Carmines. Unidimensional Scaling, pp. 7-71.

13. Measuring Health Care Cost

Gorsky, Robin D., Anne C. Haddix, and Phaedra A. Shaffer. 1996. "Cost of an Intervention." Pp. 57-75 in Anne C. Haddix, Steven M. Teutsch, Phaedra A. Shaffer, and Diane O. Dunet (Eds.), *Prevention Effectiveness: A Guide to Decision Analysis and Economic Evaluation*. New York: Oxford University Press.

*Ginsburg, Paul B., and Jeremy D. Pickreign. 1996. "Tracking Health Care Costs." *Health Affairs* 15: 140-149.

Brooten, Dorothy. 1997. "Methodological Issues Linking Costs and Outcomes." *Medical Care* 35: NS87-NS95.

Cohen, Joel W., Alan C. Monheit, Karen M. Beauregard, Steven B. Cohen, Doris C. Lefkowitz, D.E.B. Potter, John P. Sommers, Amy K. Taylor, and Ross H. Arnett, III. 1996. "The Medical Expenditure Panel Survey: A National Health Information Resource." *Inquiry* 33: 373-389.

*Dranove, David. 1995. "Measuring Cost." Pp. 61-75 in Frank A. Sloan (Ed.), *Valuing Health Care*. Cambridge, England: Cambridge University Press.

*Finkler, Steven A., James R. Knickman, Gerry Hendrickson, Mack Lipkin, Jr., and Warren G. Thompson. 1993. "A Comparison of Work-Sampling and Time-and-Motion Techniques for Studies in Health Services Research." *Health Services Research* 28: 577-597.

14. Measuring Quality of Care

*Donabedian, Avedis. 1988. "Quality Assessment and Assurance: Unity of Purpose, Diversity of Means." *Inquiry* 25: 173-192.

Brook, Robert H., Elizabeth A. McGlynn, and Paul D. Cleary. 1996. "Measuring Quality of Care." *New England Journal of Medicine* 335: 966-969.

Epstein, Arnold. 1995. "Performance Reports on Quality – Prototypes, Problems, and Prospects." *New England Journal of Medicine* 333: 57-61.

*McGlynn, Elizabeth A. 1997. "Six Challenges In Measuring The Quality of Health Care." *Health Affairs* 16: 7-21.

*Donabedian, Avedis, John R. C. Wheeler, and Leon Wyszewianski. 1982. "Quality, Cost, and Health: An Integrative Model." *Medical Care* 20: 975-992.

*Cleary, Paul D., and Susan Edgman-Levitan. 1997. "Health Care Quality: Incorporating Consumer Perspective." *JAMA* 278: 1608-1614.

*Flood, Ann Barry. 1994. "The Impact of Organizational and Managerial Factors on the Quality of Care in Health Care Organizations." *Medical Care Review* 51: 381-428.

Iezzoni, Lisa I. 1995. "Risk Adjustment for Medical Effectiveness Research: An Overview of Conceptual and Methodological Considerations." *Journal of Investigative Medicine* 43: 136-150.

*Newhouse, Joseph P. 1998. "Risk Adjustment: Where Are We Now?" *Inquiry* 35: 122-131.

*Iezzoni, Lisa I. 1997. "The Risks of Risk Adjustment." *JAMA* 278: 1600-1607.

*Landon, Bruce, Lisa I. Iezzoni, Arlene S. Ash, Michael Shwartz, Jennifer Daley, John S. Hughes, and Yevgenia D. Mackiernan. 1996. "Judging Hospitals by Severity-Adjusted Mortality Rates: The Case of CABG Surgery." *Inquiry* 33: 155-166.

*Iezzoni, Lisa I. 1997. "How Much Are We Willing To Pay for Information about Quality of Care?" *Annals of Internal Medicine* 126: 391-393.

15. Measuring Hospital Competition

Luft, Harold S., and Susan C. Maerki. 1984/85. "Competitive Potential of Hospitals and their Neighbors." *Contemporary Policy Issues* 3: 89-102.

Zwanziger, Jack, Glenn A. Melnick, and Joyce M. Mann. 1990. "Measures of Hospital Market Structure: A Review of the Alternatives and A Proposed Approach." *Socio-Economic Planning Science* 24: 81-95.

*Dranove, David, Mark Shanley, and Carol Simon. 1992. "Is Hospital Competition Wasteful?" *RAND Journal of Economics* 23: 247-62.

*Goody, Brigid. 1993. "Defining Rural Hospital Markets." *Health Services Research* 28: 183-200.

*Manheim, Larry M., Gloria J. Bazzoli, and Min-Woong Sohn. 1994. "Local Hospital Competition in Large Metropolitan Areas." *Journal of Economics & Management Strategy* 3: 143-167.

Sohn, Min-Woong. "Network Approach to Measuring Competition in the Hospital Markets." (To be distributed in class)

*Robinson, James C., and Harold S. Luft. 1985. "The Impact of Hospital Market Structure on Patient Volume, Average Length of Stay, and the Cost of Care." *Journal of Health Economics* 4: 333-356.

*Zwanziger, Jack, Glenn A. Melnick, and Kathleen M. Eyre. 1994. "Hospitals and Antitrust: Defining Markets, Setting Standards." *Journal of Health Politics, Policy, and Law* 19: 423-447.

*Melnick, Glenn A., Jack Zwanziger, Anil Bamezai, and Robert Pattison. 1992. "The Effects of Market Structure and Bargaining Position on Hospital Prices." *Journal of Health Economics* 11: 217-233.

V. INFERENTIAL METHODS

16.   Sampling and Sample Designs

Shi. Chapter 11: Sampling in Health Services Research.

*Sudman, Seymour. 1983. "Applied Sampling." Pp. 145-194 in Peter H. Rossi, James D. Wright, and Andy B. Anderson (Eds.), *Handbook of Survey Research*. San Diego, CA: Academic Press.

Cohen, Jacob. 1992. "A Power Primer." *Psychology Bulletin* 112: 155-159.

17.   Hypothesis Testing

Hempel. Chapter 3: The Test of a Hypothesis: Its Logic and Its Force.

*Kaplan. Chapter 6: Statistics.

Borenstein, Michael. 1997. "Hypothesis testing and effect size estimation in clinical trials." *Annals of Allergy, Asthma, and Immunology* 78: 5-11.

*Meehl, Paul E. 1978. "Theoretical Risks and Tabular Asterisks: Sir Karl, Sir Ronald, and the Slow Progress of Soft Psychology." *Journal of Consulting and Clinical Psychology* 46: 806-834.

*Feinstein, Alvan R. 1975. "The other side of 'statistical significance': alpha, beta, delta, and the calculation of sample size." *Clinical Pharmacology and Therapeutics* 18: 491-505.

University of Chicago
School of Social Service Administration
Chicago, IL

Course Title: Issues in Maternal and Child Health (SSA 423)
Spring 1997

Course Instructor: Sarah Lickey

DESCRIPTION

This course surveys the interdisciplinary field of maternal and child health (MCH) and presents background knowledge for social work in contemporary MCH settings. Issues in MCH policy, administration, clinical intervention, and research will be covered. The course organization parallels the cyclical nature of family development, beginning and ending with the constants of human sexuality and fertility. Issue analysis and class discussion will be informed by bio-psycho-social public health and general systems theories. Special attention will be given to: (1) MCH service design, accessibility, and patterns of use, and (2) the realities and consequences of racial, cultural, and economic diversity among MCH client populations, clinicians, administrators, and policymakers.

OBJECTIVES

A. To acquaint students with the health needs and problems of women of reproductive age, infants, children, and adolescents.

B. To familiarize students with the history and current status of major private and public MCH-related programs and policies.

C. To introduce students to social work roles in the interdisciplinary MCH field.

D. To acquaint students with theory, forms of reasoning, and value systems frequently used in guiding MCH social work service design and delivery.

TEXTS

Reading Packets

A total of 3 packets will be made available over the course of the quarter.

Supplemental Texts (SSA Reserve)

Combs-Orme, T. (1990). *Social work in maternal and child health.* New York: Springer.

Department of Health and Human Services (DHHS). (1992). *Maternal drug abuse and drug-exposed children: Understanding the problem.* Washington, DC: Author.

DHHS, Public Health Service, Substance Abuse and Mental Health Services Administration, Center for Substance Abuse Treatment. Treatment Improvement (TIP) Series.

> #5, Improving Treatment for Drug-exposed Infants

> #2, Pregnant Substance Abusing Women

Rosenfeld, L. R. (1994). *Your child and health care: A "dollars & sense" guide for families with special needs.* Baltimore, MD: Paul H. Brookes.

Wallace, H. M., Nelson, R. P., & Sweeney, P. J. (Eds.). *Maternal and child health practices* (4th ed.). Oakland, CA: Third Party.

ASSIGNMENTS

- Weekly readings & in-class discussion
- Reading summaries (lead by 3 pairs of students each week)
- Brief in-class presentation (paper summary)
- 15–20 page term paper

Reading Summaries

For 2–3 designated readings each week, pairs of students will:

- Summarize main points/findings
- Summarize epistemology
- Discuss how main points or findings: (a) fit into bio-psycho-social framework, (b) reflect MCH goals of prevention, harm reduction, or cure, and (c) may be useful to clinical, administrative, or policy MCH practitioners

Term Paper

Topic Options: Perinatal HIV testing
                       Diabetes
                       Epilepsy
                       Child sexual abuse
                       Mental retardation

   Students will show understanding and ability to apply main themes of the course to one of the above topics.

   Paper outlines will be presented in class for peer feedback during last week of the quarter.

   Final papers will be due June 11. Length: approximately 15 pages.

   Content: Use one MCH topic or problem area to:

A. Demonstrate your understanding of the major themes discussed in class (e.g., differing MCH concerns and goals, and consequences of intervention at different developmental stages; integration of services; influence of values on service design and delivery; etc.).

B. Demonstrate your understanding of concepts of primary, secondary, and tertiary prevention.

C. Demonstrate your understanding of service system issues such as access, utilization, design, & quality.

D. Address possible roles for clinical, administrative, or policy-level social work intervention.

GRADING

Term Paper—60%
Class participation—40%

COURSE PLAN

Week 1 Background Reading on Your Own

Week 2 Introductions
Course Overview
   MCH Domain
   MCH Service Goals & Indicators of Success
   MCH Service System Issues Introduction
   Theoretical Approaches to MCH Practice and Research

Week 3 Fertility, Contraception, & STDs
Unintended Pregnancy & Pregnancy Options
   Abortion & Adoption
   Infertility

Week 4 Pregnancy & the Perinatal Period I
   Risk assessment & service matching
   Genetic counseling
   Maternal outcomes

Week 5 Pregnancy & the Perinatal Period II
   Drug use in the perinatal period
   Infant outcomes: low birth weight & prematurity
   Sudden Infant Death Syndrome (SIDS)
   Perinatal loss

Week 6 Childhood I
   Breast-feeding
   Normal development & health maintenance
   Immunizations
   EPSDT

Week 7 Childhood II
   Failure to Thrive
   Children with disabilities & chronic illness, their parents, and their families
   Abuse & neglect

Week 8 Adolescent Health
   Health Maintenance & risk reduction
   "Social morbidities"

Week 9   MCH & Mental Health

> Mental illness, pregnancy & parenting
>
> Child and adolescent emotional and behavioral disorders
>
> MCH consequences of exposure to violence

Week 10 Bringing It All Together

> History of MCH Social Work—How far have we really come?
>
> Student Topical Presentations

DETAILED SCHEDULE

Week 1—No Class

Week 2— Introductions, Course Overview
Terminology, MCHB Summary Sheets, Time Line

Lesser, A. J. (1985). The origin and development of maternal and child health programs in the United States. *American Journal of Public Health, 75*(6), 590-598.

Addams, J. (1910). *Twenty Years at Hull House.* Chapter 13, pp. 200-218.

Wallace, H. M. (1994). Overview of maternal and child health around the world. In Wallace, Nelson, & Sweeney, *Maternal and child health practices* (pp. 767-798).

Marteau, T. M. Health beliefs and attributions. 1-23.

Week 3A: Fertility, Family Planning, & STDs
Lande, R. (1993). Controlling sexually transmitted diseases. In *Population reports* (Series L, No. 9). Baltimore, MD: Johns Hopkins School of Public Health, Population Information Program.

World Health Organization. (1992). *Female sterilization: A guide to provision of services.* Geneva: Author. Chapters 1, 6, 7.

Benagiano, G., & Cottingham, J. (1997). Contraceptive methods: Potential for abuse. *International Journal of Gynecology and Obstetrics, 56,* 39-46.

Gehlert, S., & Lickey, S. (1995). Social and health policy concerns raised by the introduction of the contraceptive Norplant. *Social Service Review,* 324.

Forrest, J. D. (1994). Epidemiology of unintended pregnancy and contraceptive use. *American Journal of Obstetrics and Gynecology,* 1485-1488.

Edwards, S. R. (1994). The role of men in contraceptive decision-making: Current knowledge and future implications. *Family Planning Perspectives, 26*(2), 77-82.

Optional

Snow, L. F. (1993). *Walkin' over medicine.* Boulder CO: Westview. Chapter 7, pp. 145-169.

Henshaw, S. K., & Torres, A. (1994). Family planning agencies: Services, policies and funding. *Family Planning Perspectives, 26*(2), 52-59.

Week 3B: Abortion, Adoption, & Infertility
PPFA (1996). a) Abortion pp. 1-6,

> b) D & C pp. 178-180.

c) Adoption pp. 16-20

d) Infertility pp. 231-237.

Bullough, V. L., & Bullough, B. (1995). Abortion. In V. L. Bullough & B. Bullough (Eds.), *Sexual attitudes: Myths and realities* (pp. 147-158). Amherst, NY: Prometheus.

Henshaw, S. K., & Kost, K. (1992). Parental involvement in minor's abortion decisions. *Family Planning Perspectives, 24*(5).

Sharpe, R. (1990). "She died because of a law": A mother denounces parental consent. *Ms., 1*(1), 80-81.

Editors. (1994). Program spotlight: Abortion agency offers adoption services. *Family Planning Perspectives, 25*(4), 224-225.

Lerner, S. (1996). The price of eggs: Undercover in the infertility industry. *Ms., 6*(5), 28-32, 34.

Kolata, G. (1997, March 16). Surplus of human embryos is the fruit of doctors' labor. *New York Times*, pp. A1, A14.

Recommended
Garner, C. (1995). Infertility. In C. I. Fogel & N. F. Woods, *Women's health care* (pp. 611-628). Thousand Oaks, CA: Sage.

Week 4—Pregnancy & the Perinatal Period I
Stewart, G. K. (1994). The importance of preconceptional and prenatal care. In Wallace, Nelson, & Sweeney, *Maternal and child health practices* (pp. 228-235).

Enkin, M. W. (1994). Risk in pregnancy: The reality, the perception, and the concept. *Birth, 21*(3), 131-134.

Poole, D. L., & Carlton, T. O. (1986). A model for analyzing utilization of maternal and child health services. *Health and Social Work*, 209-222.

Bedics, B. C. (1994). Nonuse of prenatal care: Implications for social work involvement. *Health and Social Work, 19*(2), 84-92.

Rauch, J. B. Social work and the genetics revolution: Genetic services. *Social Work*, 389-395.

Purdy, A. M. (1996). Genetics and reproductive risk: Can having children be immoral? In *Reproducing persons: Issues in feminist bioethics*. Ithaca, NY: Cornell University Press.

Hershey, L. (1994). Choosing disability. *Ms., 4*(4), 26-32.

Gold, E. M. (1994). Maternal mortality and reproductive mortality. In Wallace, Nelson, & Sweeney, *Maternal and child health practices* (pp. 214-220).

Week 5—Pregnancy and the Perinatal Period II
Doweiko, H. E. (1996). Chemicals and the neonate: The consequences of drug use during pregnancy. In *Concepts of chemical dependency* (3rd ed.) (Ch. 20). Pacific Grove, CA: Brooks/Cole.

The Center for Reproductive Law and Policy. (1993). *Punishing women for their behavior during pregnancy: A public health disaster*. New York: Author.

Finkelstein, N. (1994). Treatment issues for alcohol-and drug-dependent pregnant and parenting women. *Social Work, 19*(1), 7-15.

Hobel, C. (1996). Prevention of prematurity. *Pediatric Annals, 25*(4), 188-198

Long, S. H., Marquis, S., & Harrison, E. R. (1994). The costs and financing of perinatal care in the United States. *American Journal of Public Health, 84*(9), 1473-1478.

McCormick, M. C., & Lee, S. K. (1994). Estimating the costs of pregnancy-related care. *American Journal of Public Health, 84*(9), 1376.

Rowley, D., & Tosteson, H. (1993). Racial differences in preterm delivery: Developing a new paradigm. *American Journal of Preventive Medicine, 9*(6).

Pauw, M. (1991). The social worker's role with a fetal demise and stillbirth. *Health and Social Work, 16*(4), 291-297.

Douglas, A. (1997, March 16). Walking through the fire: A journey of joy and hope becomes one of pain and grief. *Chicago Tribune*, Section 13, pp. 1, 2, 6.

Goldberg, J. (1996, September). Should dying babies be organ donors? *Redbook*, pp. 132-135, 154.

Week 6—Childhood I

WHO/UNICEF. (1989). *Protecting, promoting, and supporting breast-feeding: The special role of maternity services.* Geneva: World Health Organization.

Nash, J. M. (1997, February 3). Fertile minds. *Time*, pp. 48-56.

Other readings TBA

Week 7—Childhood II

NRCCAN. (1995). *Maltreatment of children with disabilities: Information sheet.* Englewood, CO: National Resource Center on Child Abuse and Neglect.

Nash, K. B. (1994). Introduction. In K. B. Nash (Ed.), *Psychosocial aspects of sickle cell disease: Past, present, and future directions of research* (pp. 1-6). Binghamton, NY: Haworth.

Holbrook, C. T., & Phillips, G. (1994). Natural history of sickle cell disease and the effects on biopsychosocial development. In K. B. Nash (Ed.), *Psychosocial aspects of sickle cell disease: Past, present, and future directions of research* (pp. 7-18). Binghamton, NY: Haworth.

Bradley, R. H., Parette, H. P., & VanBiervliet, A. (1995). Families of young technology-dependent children and the social worker. In R. B. Smith & H. G. Clinton (Eds.), *Social work in pediatrics* (pp. 23-37). Binghamton, NY: Haworth.

Brown, D. G., Krieg, K., & Belluck, F. (1995). A model for group intervention with the chronically ill: Cystic fibrosis and the family. In R. B. Smith & H. G. Clinton (Eds.), *Social work in pediatrics* (pp. 81-94). Binghamton, NY: Haworth.

Horst, M. L. (1995). Model for management of services to low income pediatric asthma patients. In R. B. Smith & H. G. Clinton (Eds.), *Social work in pediatrics* (pp. 81-94). Binghamton, NY: Haworth.

Week 8—Adolescent Health

MMWR Vol. 45. No. SS-4. Youth Risk Behavior Surveillance—United States, 1995.

Raphael, D. (1996). Determinants of health of North American adolescents: Evolving definitions, recent findings, and proposed research agenda. *Journal of Adolescent Health, 19*(1), 6-16.

Santelli, J., Morreale, M., Wigton, A., & Grason, H. (1996). School health centers and primary care for adolescents: A review of the literature. *Journal of Adolescent Health, 18*(5), 357-366.

Ray, J., & Roloff, M. (1994). Schooling for young street mothers and their babies. *Children Today, 23*(2), 29-31

Brooks-Gunn, & Paikoff, R. L. (1993). Sex is a gamble and kissing is a game: Adolescent sexuality and health promotion. In S. G. Millstein, A. C. Petersen, & E. O. Nightingale (Eds.), *Promoting the health of adolescents: New directions for the twenty-first century* (Ch. 9). New York: Oxford University Press.

Earls, F., Cairns, R. B., & Mercy, J. A. (1993). The control of violence and the promotion of nonviolence in adolescents. In S. G. Millstein, A. C. Petersen, & E. O. Nightingale (Eds),

Promoting the health of adolescents: New directions for the twenty-first century (Ch. 13). New York: Oxford University Press.

Grossman, J., & Cotes, C. (1996). Suicide morbidity and mortality in Latina Youth: Prevention opportunities. In B. J. McElmurry & R. S. Parker (Eds.), *Annual review of women's health* (Vol. 3, Ch. 10). New York: National League for Nursing Press.

Week 9—MCH & Mental Health
Reference Materials
Federation for Families for Children's Mental Health. (1995). *Collaborations: Building partnerships.*

Assigned Readings
Mowbray, C. T., Oyserman, D., Zemencuk, J. K., & Ross, S. R. (1995). Motherhood for women with serious mental illness: Pregnancy, childbirth, and the postpartum period. *American Journal of Orthopsychiatry, 65*(1), 21-38.

Marsh, D. T. (1996). Families of children and adolescents with serious emotional disturbance: Innovations in theory, research, and practice. In C.A. Heflinger & C.T. Nixon (Eds.), *Families and the mental health system for children and adolescents: Policy, services, and research* (Ch. 5). Thousand Oaks, CA: Sage.

Osofsky, J. D. (1995). The effects of exposure to violence on young children. *American Psychologist, 50*(9), 782-788.

Goleman, D. Early violence leaves its mark on the brain. *New York Times.*

Bagley, C. (1995). Early sexual experience and sexual victimization of children and adolescents: Review and summary. In *Child Sexual Abuse and Mental Health in Adolescents and Adults: British and Canadian Perspectives* (Ch. 9). Avebury.

Additional Reading
Modrcin, M. J., & Robison, J. (1991). Parents of children with emotional disorders: Issues for consideration and practice. *Community Mental Health Journal, 27*(4), 281-292.

Roberts, M. C. (Ed.). (1996). *Model programs in child and family mental health.* Mahway, NJ: Lawrence Erlbaum.

American Orthopsychiatric Association. (1994). Strengthening mental health in Head Start: Pathways to quality improvement [Report of the Task Force on Head Start and Mental Health]. New York: Author.

Petr, C. G., & Spano, R. N. (1990). Evolution of social services for children with emotional disorders. *Social Work, 35,* 228-234.

Week 10—Bringing It All Together
See history readings for Week 1
Review of readings throughout quarter

Additional Readings
Mahowald, M. B. (1993). *Women and children in health care: An unequal majority.* New York: Oxford University Press.

Craft, A., & Craft, M. (1983). *Sex education and counseling for mentally handicapped people.* Baltimore, MD: University Park Press.

Feinstein, J. S. (1993). The relationship between socioeconomic status and health: A review of the literature. *Milbank Quarterly, 71*(2), 279-322.

Glanz, K., Lewis, F. M., & Rimer, B. K. (Eds.). (1990). *Health behavior and health education: Theory and research and practice.* San Francisco: Jossey-Bass.

Fogel, C. I., & Woods, C. F. (1995). *Women's health care: A comprehensive handbook.* Thousand Oaks, CA: Sage.

Maternal and Child Health Bureau. (1995). *Public MCH program functions: Essential public health services to promote maternal and child health in America.*

Millstein, S. G., Petersen, A. C., & Nightingale, E. O. (Eds.). (1993). *Promoting the health of adolescents: New directions for the twenty-first century.* New York: Oxford University Press.

Musick, J. S. (1993). *Young, poor, and pregnant: The psychology of teenage motherhood.* New Haven, CT: Yale University Press.

Rolland, J. S. (1995). Mastering family challenges in serious illness and disability. In F. Walsh (Ed.), *Normal family processes* (2nd ed., pp. 444-473). New York: Guilford.

Schild, S., & Black, R. B. (1984). *Social work and genetics: A guide for practice.* Binghamton, NY: Haworth.

University of Chicago
School of Social Service Administration
Chicago, IL

Course Title: Urban Health Care (SSA 487)
Spring Quarter 1998

Course Instructors: Cheryl Rucker-Whitaker, Richard H. Sewell, & James Unland

DESCRIPTION

This course will examine the health problems of people who live in large metropolitan areas and the political economy of urban health care delivery. A special focus on alternative uses of tax dollars to serve the medically indigent population of Cook County will be the core consideration in the course. Many cities like Chicago are experiencing an increase of AIDS, TB, substance abuse, and the exacerbation of social pathologies such as violence and homelessness. At the same time, health care provider structures and arrangements are changing which place additional strains on public sector health systems. The alternatives available to large cities to these challenges and the relative influence of their own urban economies upon that response will be discussed and analyzed.

Each class will be devoted to discussion and analysis of the specific topics indicated in advance for that class. The course will be conducted primarily in a seminar format, which requires that each student come to class prepared to participate in discussions.

GRADING AND ASSIGNMENTS

Grades will be determined using the following criteria:

Final Paper	40%
Problem Sets	55%
Class Participation	5%

Final Paper

The final paper will test students' understanding of and ability to apply the theories and concepts from the readings and class discussions. Students will also have the opportunity to submit their final papers for publication in the *Journal of Health Care Finance*. The objectives of the paper are:

- to foster the integration of the materials studied in the course;

- to encourage students to develop their own ideas, opinions, and reactions regarding these materials;

- to improve students' writing, reasoning, and analytic skills;

- to provide solid evidence of what students have learned from the course; and

- to challenge students to be creative problem-solvers.

Problem Sets

Five problem sets will be completed by each student as if composed by a senior policy advisor. Some of these problem sets will require the use of spreadsheets and data analysis. The problem sets will address the topics assigned and will provide the basis for writing the final paper.

Class Participation

The class participation grade will be based upon the quality of thinking and insights reflected in students' comments and questions and not necessarily upon the volume or frequency of participation. Students will be expected to discuss the ideas and concepts in the readings and the lectures in the context of the urban health system structure, the major problems, and alternative solutions and reform strategies.

Reading assignments will be required in preparation for each class. Class discussion will focus on the major readings. Optional readings may be suggested from time to time which will provide students with broader and more detailed insights into the assigned topics.

TEXTS

Required

Abraham, L. K. (1993). *Mama Might Be Better Off Dead: The Failure of Health Care in Urban America.* Chicago: University of Chicago Press.

This book may be purchased from the Seminary Co-op Bookstore. A packet of readings will also be sold.

Optional

Brecher, C., & Spiezio, S. (1995). *Privatization and Public Hospitals: Choosing Wisely for New York City.* New York: Twentieth Century Fund Press.

Ginzberg, E., Berliner, H., & Ostow, M. (1997). *Improving Health Care of the Poor: The New York City Experience.* New Brunswick, NJ: Transaction.

Aday, L. A. (1993). *At Risk in America: The Health and Health Care Needs of Vulnerable Populations in the United States.* San Francisco: Jossey-Bass.

Braithwaite, R. L., & Taylor, S. E. (Eds.). (1992). *Health Issues in the Black Community.* San Francisco: Jossey-Bass.

CLASS SCHEDULE

Session 1 Health and Medicine

Introduction to Urban Health Problems

Lecturer: Rucker-Whitaker

Readings:

Whiteis, D. G., & Salmon, J. W. (1992). Public Health Care Delivery Systems in Five U.S. Municipalities: Lessons and Implications. *Henry Ford Hospital Medical Journal, 40*(1 & 2), 16-25.

Abraham, L. K. *Mama Might Be Better Off Dead: The Failure of Health Care in Urban America.*

Fossett, J. W., & Perloff, J. D. (1995, December). *The "New" Health Reform and Access to Care: The Problem of the Inner City* [prepared for The Kaiser Commission on the Future of Medicaid]. Washington, DC: Kaiser Family Foundation.

Session 2   Public Health in Chicago and Cook County

The Cook County Bureau of Health Services

Lecturer: Sewell

Readings:

Metropolitan Planning Council. (1993, June). *Public Health: The Best Kept Secret.* Chicago: Author.

Collection of information from Cook County 1988 Executive Budget Recommendations:

1998 Cook County Organizational Chart

- Overview of Cook County Health Facilities, E155-E158
- Bureau of Health Measurable Goals (overview), L1-3
- Bureau of Health Services Organizational Chart, L4
- Department summaries and specific measurable goals for the Bureau of Health, Cermak Health Services, Provident Hospital, Ambulatory and Community Health Network of Cook County, Department of Public Health, Cook County Hospital, Oak Forest Hospital, Health Fund and Managed Care Support Fund, various pages between L10 and L144

Collection of information from the 1998 Executive Budget Recommendations Revenue Estimate:

- Fiscal Year 1998 Estimated Revenues and Other Resources, p. 2-3
- Fiscal Year 1998 County Health Fund Estimated Revenues and Other Resources, p. 6
- Table 16: Patient Fees for the Health Fund, 1994-1998, p. 54
- Table 27: Revenues for the Health Fund, 1994-1998, p. 59

Hinz, G. (1998, Feb. 9). A hospital plan that defied odds. *Crain's Chicago Business*, p. 1

Problem Set One: Basic trends in revenues, average length of stay and patient days. (Due Session 4)

Session 3   Urban Policy Analysis

Lecturer: Edward F. Lawlor, University of Chicago

Readings:

Peterson, P. (1981). The Three Policy Arenas. In *City Limits* (pp. 41-65). Chicago: University of Chicago Press.

Jargowsky, P., & Bane, M. (1990). Ghetto Poverty: Basic Questions. In L. Lynn & M. McGeary (Eds.), *Inner-City Poverty in the United States.* Washington, DC: National Academy Press.

Session 4   Trends in Modern Health Care Delivery in the U.S.

Trends in Serving the Medically Indigent

Population-Based Health Care Management

Lecturer: Unland

Readings:

Gaskin, D. J. (1997). The Impact of Health Maintenance Organization Penetration on the Use of Hospitals that Serve Minority Communities. *Medical Care, 35*(12), 1190-1203.

Lipson, D. J., & Naierman, N. (1996). Effects of Health Systems Changes on Safety-Net Providers. *Health Affairs, 15*(2), 33-48.

Mitchell, M. K. (1996, Dec. 2). Critics of Privatizing N.Y. Hospital Miss Its Promise. *Modern Healthcare, 26*(49).

Goldman, J. J., & Perry, T. (1995, Nov. 2). Code Blue: The Crisis in Los Angeles County Health Care. *Los Angeles Times*, p. A1.

"Poverty, Illness and the Future of Cook County Hospital," a working draft prepared for the Task Force of Health Care for the Poor, a joint project of Center for Urban Research and Policy Studies, the University of Chicago and Metropolitan Planning Council, April 1986.

Session 5   Review of Conclusions of Prior Studies of the Need for a New Cook County Hospital

Lecturer: Unland

Readings:

Bobrow, Thomas, and associates. (1994, Jan. 20). *Feasibility Study Report—Part I.* Chicago: Author.

Bobrow, Thomas, and associates. (1994, May). *Feasibility Study Report—Part II.* Chicago: Author.

Coopers and Lybrand. (1993, November). *Cook County Bureau of Health Services Advisory Committee: Preliminary Financial Projections for a New Cook County Hospital.* Chicago: Author.

Illinois Health Facilities Planning Board. "Certificate of Need Staff Analysis, July 1993, General Review Criteria: Alternatives to the Proposed Project," Attachment 14, p. 23-40.

Most Common Questions About the New Cook County Hospital, April 1997.

Problem Set Two: Review the feasibility studies and the certificate of need materials and prepare a criticism of the alternatives available to the County in replacing Cook County Hospital and the pros and cons associated with each alternative. Compare Cook County's role to at least three other public sector health systems (due April 21).

Session 6   Cook County Hospital's Service Areas and Scope of Services

Lecturer: Unland

Readings:

Starr, P. (1982). The Coming of the Corporation. In *The Social Transformation of American Medicine* (pp. 420-449). New York: Basic Books.

Illinois Health Facilities Planning Board. "Certificate of Need Staff Analysis, July 1993, General Review Criteria: Alternatives to the Proposed Project," Attachment 14, p. 23-40.

Session 7   Comparison of Medical Services by Service Category Between Cook County Hospital and Community Hospitals

Lecturer: Sewell

Readings:

Illinois Health Facilities Planning Board. Certificate of Need Staff Analysis, July 1993, City of Chicago Short-Term General Hospitals by Community Area, Attachment 10, p. 13.

Problem Set Three: Prepare a market share analysis by payor category, geography, and service category for Cook County Hospital's major services (due April 28).

Session 8   Analysis of Capacity and Capabilities of Community Hospitals

Lecturer: Sewell

Session 9 Measuring the Funding Gap: Per Diem and Per Unit Comparisons Between Cook County and the Private Sector

Lecturer: Unland

Problem Set Four: Compare costs and rates for all major Cook County services (due May 5).

Session 10 The Socioeconomics of Access to Care

Lecturer: Sewell

Readings:

Children's Health: Is Insurance a Panacea? (1997, Spring). *Rand Research Review, 21*(1), p. 6-7.

Pappas, G., Hadden, W. C., Kozak, L. J., & Fisher, G. F. (1997). Potentially Avoidable Hospitalizations: Inequalities in Rates Between U.S. Socioeconomic Groups. *American Journal of Public Health, 87*(5), 811-816.

Grumback, L., Vranizan, K., & Bindman, A. B. (1997). Physician Supply and Access to Care in Urban Communities. *Health Affairs,* 16(1), 71-86.

Komaromy, M., Lurie, N., & Bindman, A. B. (1995). California Physician's Willingness to Care for the Poor. *Western Journal of Medicine, 162*(2), 127-132.

Session 11 The Socioeconomics of Health: Race and Class

Lecturer: Rucker-Whitaker

Readings:

Feinstein, J. S. (1993). The Relationship Between Socioeconomic Status and Health: A Review of the Literature. *Milbank Quarterly, 71*(2), 279-321.

Adler, N. E., Boyce, T., Chesney, M. A., Folkman, S., & Syme, S. L. (1993). Socioeconomic Inequalities in Health: No Easy Solution. *Journal of the American Medical Association, 269*(24), 3140-3145.

McCord, C., & Freeman, H. P. (1990). Excess Mortality in Harlem. *New England Journal of Medicine, 322*(3), 173-177.

Sorlie, P. D., Backlund, E., & Keller, J. B. (1995). U.S. Mortality by Economic, Demographic and Social Characteristics: The National Longitudinal Mortality Study. *American Journal of Public Health, 85*(7), 949-956.

Session 12 Medicaid

Lecturer: Henry Webber, University of Chicago

Readings:

Joseph, L. B., & Webber, H. S. (1985). Medicaid Myths and Realities: An Analysis of the Illinois Medicaid Program, 1983-1994. Unpublished manuscript.

Rowland, D., Rosenbaum, S., Simon, L., & Chait, E. (1995, March). Medicaid and Managed Care: Lessons from the Literature (a report of the Kaiser Commission on the Future on Medicaid. Menlo Park, CA: The Henry J. Kaiser Family Foundation.

Rosenbaum, S., & Dievler, A. (1993, February). *Providing Primary Health Care to Medicaid Beneficiaries: Key Elements of Effective Programs.* Washington, DC: Kaiser Commission on the Future of Medicaid.

Session 13 The Role of the State of Illinois in Expanding Medicaid Enrollment
   The Uninsured in Illinois and Cook County

Lecturer: Michael Gelder, Consultant

Readings:

Lipson, D. J., & Schrodel, S. P. (1996). *State Initiatives in Health Care Reform: State Subsidized Insurance Programs for Low-Income People.* Washington, DC: Alpha Center.

Illinois Department of Public Aid. (1998, March 6). *Illinois Medical Assistance Program and KidCare: Request for Proposals from Health Maintenance Organizations.* pp. i-iv, 1-5, 25-26, 56-58. [entire document can be found at the Illinois Department of Public Aid's Web page at http://www.state.il.us/dpa/rfp.htm]

Session 14 Exploring Various Levels of Private Sector Contracting by the County: Sensitivity Analysis

Lecturer: Unland

Problem Set Five: Prepare a sensitivity analysis of using a private sector contracting arrangement as an alternative to a replacement hospital. Estimate the cost savings and discuss the expected negative consequences (due May 21).

Session 15 The Spread of AIDS and Sexually Transmitted Diseases in Urban Communities

Lecturer: Supriya Madhaven, Chicago Department of Public Health

Readings:

Jenkins, B. (1992). AIDS/HIV Epidemics in the Black Community. In R. L. Braithwaite & S. E. Taylor (Eds.), Health issues in the Black community, pp. 55-63. San Francisco: Jossey-Bass.

Whitman, S., & Murphy, J. (1997, Sept. 19). *Description of the Recent Decline in Chicago's AIDS Mortality, September 1997.* Information presented at the Chicago Health Policy Research Council's Downtown Health Policy Series.

Sikkema, K. J., et al. (1996). HIV Risk Behaviors among Women Living in Low-Income, Inner-City Housing Developments. *American Journal of Public Health, 86*(8), 1123-1128.

Session 16 Environmental Health Issues: Lead and Asthma

Lecturer: Linda Murray, Cook County Bureau of Health Services

Readings:

Weiss, K. B., Gergen, P. J., & Crain, E. F. (1992). Inner-city Asthma: The Epidemiology of an Emerging U.S. Public Health Concern. *CHEST, 101*(6): S362-S367.

Berney, B. (1993). Round and Round it Goes: The Epidemiology of Childhood Lead Poisoning, 1950–1990. *Milbank Quarterly, 71*(1), 3.

Approaches to Solutions and Reforms

Session 17 The Fragmentation of Home Care and a Neighborhood Alternative

Lecturer: Susan Reed, DePaul University

Readings:

Benjamin, A. E. (1993). An Historical Perspective on Home Care Policy. *Milbank Quarterly, 71*(1), 129-166.

Session 18 Innovative Initiatives for the Uninsured: Access to Care

Lecturer: Victoria Bigelow, Suburban Primary Health Care Council

Readings:

Krieg, R., & Cooksey, J. (1995). *Barriers to Health Policy Implementation in Metropolitan Chicago.* Chicago: Chicago Health Policy Research Council. Unpublished manuscript.

Assignment: Turn in final paper (Spring graduates)

Session 19 Public Health and Health Care Reform: The Role of Communities

Lecturer: Sewell

Readings:

Institute of Medicine, National Academy of Sciences. (1988). A vision of public health in America: An attainable ideal. In *The future of public health* (pp. 35-55). Washington, DC: National Academy Press.

Session 20 Future Options for Cook County's Health System

Lecturer: Unland
Assignment: Turn in final paper

Syracuse University
School of Social Work
Syracuse, NY

Course Title: AIDS: Social and Preventive Issues (SWK 785)
Fall 1998

Course Instructor: Susan Taylor-Brown

OVERVIEW

This course studies policy and practice issues affecting individuals infected by human immunodeficiency virus (HIV). It examines the nature of illness, its psychosocial sequelae, the differential impact on ethnic/cultural groups in the U.S., and strategies for ethnic-sensitive practice.

DESCRIPTION

Social work has a history of responding to the needy and oppressed of society. Today, we are facing a pandemic of Acquired Immunodeficiency Syndrome (AIDS) that has major implications for social workers in every practice setting. Persons with HIV disease (PWHIV), ranging from those who are HIV+ to those who have AIDS, are experiencing discriminatory actions in almost every aspect of society, including housing, employment, law enforcement, education, and medical care.

We are beginning to understand the impact of AIDS not only on the person who has AIDS but on extended family members, significant others, and the community. The HIV virus is differentially affecting ethnic/cultural groups in the United States, and each of these groups is responding uniquely to this illness. Therefore, it is important for social workers to understand the cultural differences when planning and providing services.

This course is designed to provide in-depth knowledge about HIV disease and to produce social workers who will provide community leadership. The course will assist the student in becoming more comfortable working with individuals who are infected with HIV. The seminar will use a combination of approaches: lectures, class discussion, videotapes, presentations by community providers and individuals affected by HIV disease. The seminar will help students become more aware of: (1) the medical realities of HIV disease; (2) the psychosocial implications of the illness as related to treatment issues; (3) the policy issues relevant to the illness; (4) methods of prevention; (5) issues related to professional practice with persons who test antibody-positive to HIV; and (6) program planning issues from program design to implementation. The course will assist students to provide culturally sensitive services to individuals infected with HIV or individuals affected by HIV.

OBJECTIVES

Students will be able to:

1. Articulate the medical aspects of HIV disease and related illnesses such as tuberculosis (TB).

2. Identify the psychosocial needs of PWHIV, their significant others, and the community.

3. Articulate a plan for implementing programs for PWHIV and their significant others from prevention to post-death interventions.

4. Analyze social policies and legislation related to AIDS, particularly regarding issues of civil rights and discrimination.

5. Articulate the differential impact of HIV disease on diverse populations and the relationship of poverty to the differential incidence and prevalence rates.

6. Articulate personal values and attitudes towards AIDS and examine their relationship to professional practice.

7. Critically review quantitative and qualitative HIV studies with emphasis on the ethical issues involved when doing research with vulnerable populations.

TEXTS

Required

Aronstein, D. M., & Thompson, B. J. (Eds.). (1998). *HIV and social work: A practitioner's guide.* Binghamton, NY: Harrington Park.

Farmer, P., Connors, M., & Simmons, J. (1996). *Women, poverty and AIDS: Sex, drugs and structural violence.* Monroe, ME: Common Courage Press.

Gluck, E., & Rosenthal, E., (1995). *The effectiveness of AIDS prevention efforts: HIV prevention: State of the science.* Washington, DC: American Psychological Association.

Lynch, V. (Ed.). (1999, in press). *HIV/AIDS at year 2000: A sourcebook for social workers.* Boston: Allyn and Bacon.

Working Committee on HIV, Children and Families. (1996). *Families in crisis: Report of the working committee on HIV, children and families.* New York: Federation of Protestant Social Workers.

Wyatt-Morley, C. (1997). *AIDS memoir: Journal of an HIV-positive mother.* West Hartford, CT: Kumarian.

Recommended

Mann, J., & Tarantola, D. (1996) *AIDS in the world II.* New York: Oxford University Press.

ASSIGNMENTS AND EVALUATION PROCEDURES

A. Class Participation: Students are expected to have read the assigned readings and to participate in class discussion. Students are encouraged to consider the applicability of the readings to their practice. There will be opportunities for individual and group presentations of assignments.

B. Required Readings and Assignments:

    a. See class calendar for reading assignments.

    b. Students are expected to develop a 1-hour group presentation for the prevention unit.

    c. Students are expected to complete four written assignments: Student journal, the midterm, a research paper, and personal accounts.

Assignment 1. Student Journal/Personal Accounts

Student Journal

Students are to make journal entries that should focus on the student's reactions to either: (a) Seminar discussion; (b) The assigned readings; (c) Outside readings; (d) Class media presentations; or (e) Discussions with others about HIV infection.

Students are encouraged to critically explore their feelings about HIV infection and how their feelings influence practice.

The log will be collected at the beginning of the fourth session and due every third class thereafter. Since these papers are collected, please do not use a notebook. Students will receive written feedback from the instructor for each entry.

A total of three entries are to be submitted during the term. No late entries are accepted.

Personal Accounts

You can read either Wyatt-Morley's memoir or a personal account book of your choice. You will write a one-page reaction paper to the book you choose, identifying the key issues the person dealt with and your reactions to those issues. Finally, make a recommendation for others about whether they should read these books or not, and why. This can be submitted anytime up to Session 12.

Experiential Option

In lieu of two log entries you can volunteer eight hours at an AIDS-related agency or community-based AIDS activity, e.g., Rays of Hope, a conference addressing the needs of African Americans and Latinos in Rochester, NY. Other community conference options will be announced in class. You will write a one-page reaction paper to the experience, identifying the key issues you observed at the agency/conference and your reactions to it. Please attach either your registration or conference brochure. Instructor approval required.

Journal Due Dates: (#1) Session 3, (#2) Session 7, and (#3) Session 10.

Assignment 2. Midterm Exam

For this open-book, essay exam, you will have an opportunity to synthesize the course readings and class discussion. To prepare for the exam, it is recommended that you read and outline the assigned readings from the first class through Session 7. The essay questions will ask you to apply this reading to the questions. You must provide specific examples from the assigned readings. The Midterm exam will be given during class on Session 8.

Assignment 3. Class Presentation

For Unit IV, Prevention, students in groups of 4–6 will develop a population-specific prevention presentation that will incorporate the assigned readings for that sub-unit and the articles obtained for the final group research project. You may choose who you will work with. Students are encouraged to interview service providers to obtain a practitioner's perspective regarding the challenges of serving this population. These presentations will begin Session 12.

Assignment 4. Research Paper (Due: Session 14)

The research paper is to be an analysis of a current psychosocial issue in HIV/AIDS and will include a review of the HIV/AIDS literature (1992–present), and a thorough discussion of the policy and/or practice implications. This can be either a group paper or an individual paper.

- Each student must do a computerized literature and web search (the search must be submitted as part of your final paper), and review more than seven refereed social work journal articles (popular articles may be included as supplemental sources; however, they are *not* primary sources and cannot be included as part of the seven refereed articles).

- critical analysis must incorporate assigned readings

- 8–10 pages for individual paper; group paper length will be determined based upon the size of the group

- APA Style

Note: A detailed group project guide, paper guide and grading guideline will be distributed Session 4. Group topics should be submitted as soon as possible. They *must* be submitted by Session 9. The Research Paper is due Session 15.

Please note: no extensions will be granted.

C. Grading

Class Participation (includes 3 journal entries or 1+ experiential learning option)	20%
Midterm	30%
Research Paper	30%
Personal Account Exercise	20%

CONTENT OUTLINE

UNIT I. AIDS: DIAGNOSIS AND TREATMENT

Sessions 1 & 2

Content:

*   epidemiology of HIV infection with emphasis on the disproportionate impact on ethnic/cultural minorities

*   scientific paradigms: how much do we know?

*   at-risk behaviors vs. at-risk populations

*   disease characteristics

*   transmission: sexually transmitted diseases

*   screening tests: false positives and negatives

*   treatment modalities: protease inhibitors, vaccine trials, clinical treatment trials

*   course of illness

*   TB: the intersection of two epidemics

These sessions will combine a lecture, videotape and class discussion of the above material.

Required Readings

Aronstein & Thompson, Section I, 3-74

Lynch, Ch. 1, HIV/AIDS and Social Work: The Medical Context, 1-12

Recommended Readings (on reserve)

Mann & Tarantola, Ch.1, Global overview: A powerful HIV/AIDS pandemic, 5-40

Mann & Tarantola, Ch. 10, Treatment of HIV disease: Problems, progress and potential, 159-164

Mann & Tarantola, Ch. 11, Long-term survivors, 165-170

Mann & Tarantola, Ch. 12, HIV-2 infection: Current knowledge, 171-176

UNIT II. SOCIAL CONSTRUCTION OF AIDS

Sessions 3, 4, 5

1st Journal Assignment due: Session 4

Content:

*   stigma/discrimination

*   the impact of marginalization on PWHIV

*   the differential impact on communities of color, injecting drug users & their partners and gay men

- fear: AFRAIDS
- parental loss due to HIV
- stigma not only of patients but family and caregivers alike

Class Sessions:

A lecture will provide current information regarding the psychosocial research literature. Then the seminar group will meet with a PWHIV or a family member. The PWHIV or family member will share his/her experiences with the group, and we will examine the service implications.

Additionally, service providers who are working with infected parents will present the challenges of permanency planning.

Required Readings

Aronstein & Thompson, Section II, Part A, 75-164

Farmer, complete text: Ch. 1, Women, Poverty, and AIDS; Ch. 2, A Global Perspective; Ch. 3, Sex, Drugs, and Structural Violence; Ch. 4, Women and HIV Infection; Ch. 5, Rereading Social Services; Ch. 6, Rereading Public Health; Ch. 7, Rereading Clinical Medicine; Ch. 8, Confronting Obstacles; Ch. 9, Making Common Cause

Lynch, Ch. 2, The Psychosocial Context, 18-32

Lynch, Ch. 3, Ethical Issues and Dilemmas in HIV/AIDS, 33-49

Recommended Readings

Mann & Tarantola, Part IV, Institutional Response, Chs. 30–37, 311-426

UNIT III. CARE FOR THE PROFESSIONAL CAREGIVER
Sessions 6 & 7
2nd Journal Assignment due: Session 7
Content:
- Stigma of the professional who is associated with a stigmatized group
- Need for support
- Risk in the health care workplace
- Worker's responsibility to serve AIDS patient
- Health care team formation
- Fear
- Family pressures
- Morale
- Image
- Interdisciplinary Care: team dynamics, working with colleagues who are HIV+
- Care for the professional caregivers

Class Session: These sessions will help students to provide service to HIV-infected and -affected individuals. There are unique dynamics related to the pandemic which affect our ability to provide care.

Required Readings

Aronstein & Thompson, Section V, 527-560, Section II, Part B, 165-302, Section III, Part A, 315-386

Assessing the social work response to HIV/AIDS: A report prepared for the National Association of Social Workers Task Force on HIV/AIDS. Executive Summary. **(To be handed out in class)**

Session 8   MIDTERM EXAM

UNIT IV. PREVENTION
Sessions 9, 10, 11, 12
3rd Journal Assignment due: Session 10
Personal Account Exercise due: Session 12
Group Presentations: Sessions 10, 11, 12
Content:
- identification of high-risk behaviors
- public health models of behavior change and harm reduction (see, e.g., Prochaska, J., DiClimente, C., & Norcross, J. (1992, Sept.). In search of how people change. *American Psychologist*, 1102-1113.)
- lifestyle modification: sexual practices and IV drug use
- development of culturally sensitive prevention strategies

Class Sessions: For the first part of seminar, the instructor will review the recent literature regarding prevention efforts. Then an outreach worker will present information about his/her job and the class will have an opportunity to discuss prevention efforts in the Central New York area. Selected AIDS prevention videos will be shared.

Unit IV(a) Population-Specific Approaches
Required Readings
  Gluck & Rosenthal, Ch. 1, Office technology assessment report: The effectiveness of AIDS prevention efforts, 1-39

  Gluck & Rosenthal, Ch. 7, Application of social marketing principles to AIDS education, 276-308

  Gluck & Rosenthal, Ch. 8, Economic evaluations of HIV/AIDS education and primary prevention, 309-341

  Gluck & Rosenthal, Ch. 9, HIV education: National surveys, counseling and testing programs and the role of physicians, 342-367

  Lynch, Ch. 14, HIV/AIDS prevention, 188-196

Recommended Readings:
  Mann & Tarantola, Ch. 9, The contribution of social and behavioral science to HIV prevention, 131-158

Unit IV(b) Men Who Have Sex with Men
Required Readings
  Aronstein & Thompson, p. 411-430

  Gluck & Rosenthal, Ch. 3, Does HIV prevention work for men who have sex with men? 74-123

  Lynch, Ch. 11, Safer sex maintenance among gay men: HIV-prevention challenges and intervention strategies, 148- 164.

Recommended Readings:
  Mann & Tarantola, Ch. 22, Male homosexuality and HIV, 252-258

Unit IV(c) Adolescents and Youth
Required Readings
  Aronstein & Thompson, 387-402

  Gluck & Rosenthal, Ch. 5, A review of education programs designed to reduce sexual risk taking behaviors, 159-235

  Lynch, Ch. 9, Adolescents at risk for HIV infection: A growing concern, 123-137.

Recommended Readings
   Mann & Tarantola, Ch. 21, Youth and HIV/AIDS, 236-251
   Mann & Tarantola, Ch. 26, Pediatric HIV/AIDS, 273-277
   Mann & Tarantola, Ch. 27, Orphans, 278-286

Unit IV(d) Women
Recommended Readings
   Aronstein & Thompson, 431-442

   Gluck & Rosenthal, Ch. 6, A review of HIV interventions of at-risk women, 236-273
Recommended Readings
   Mann & Tarantola, Ch. 16 Women-controlled HIV prevention methods, 196-201

   Mann & Tarantola, Ch. 19 HIV/AIDS among women, 215-228

   Mann & Tarantola, Ch. 20 HIV in women: Gaps, 229-235

   Mann & Tarantola, Ch. 23 Sexual behavior among heterosexuals, 259-263

   Mann & Tarantola, Ch. 29 Are we learning from the lessons of the past?, 302-309

Unit IV(e) Injecting Drug Users
Required Reading
   Aronstein & Thompson, p. 303-314

   Gluck & Rosenthal, Ch. 2, HIV Prevention for Injecting Drug Users, 40-73
Recommended Readings
   Mann & Tarantola, Ch. 24, Risk reduction among injecting drug users, 264-267

   Mann & Tarantola, Ch. 25, HIV/AIDS in prisons, 268-272

Unit IV(f) African Americans, Latinos
Required Readings
   Aronstein & Thompson, p. 51-64, 443-450

   Gluck & Rosenthal, Ch. 4, Analysis of AIDS prevention among African Americans and Latinos in the
      U.S., 124-158

   Lynch, Ch. 4, HIV/AIDS issues among African Americans: Oppressed, gifted and Black, 50-65

   Lynch, Ch. 6, AIDS and women of color, 79-96

   Lynch, Ch. 7, Latinos and HIV, 97-106

UNITS V and VI. THE CONTINUUM OF CARE FOR THOSE INFECTED WITH HIV: POLICY and PRACTICE IMPLICATIONS

Sessions 13, 14, 15
Unit V. Practice
• Case management

• Prevention

• Acute care

• Long-term care

• Care for the caregivers

Unit VI. Policy Issues
• Orphans

• Needle exchange, condom distribution in high schools and in jails

- Mandatory testing and Fourth Amendment issues
- Testing of healthcare workers
- Legal issues:
    - Risks and responsibilities
    - Labor law and liability
- AIDS Commissions: Presidential, Congressional
- Funding Issues
- Agency Policies
- Ethical Issues

Class Session: The last two units will combine key policy issues with treatment issues. Various community providers will share their experiences with the seminar.

Required Readings

Aronstein & Thompson, 483-510

Lynch, Ch. 5, Parents and their children: Planning in the face of uncertainty, 66-78

Lynch, Ch. 8, Social work treatment with caregivers: Taking care of them so they can take care of their loved ones, 107- 122

Lynch, Ch. 10, HIV and later life, 138-147

Lynch, Ch. 12, The dual challenges of HIV and drug use: What to know, what to do, 165-177

Lynch, Ch. 13, Common concerns: Social and psychological issues for persons with HIV, 178-187

Lynch, Ch. 15, Advocacy and social policy issues, 197-210

Lynch, Ch. 16, Adherence to treatment as social work challenges, 211-227

Lynch, Ch. 17, Mental health issues in HIV disease, 228-241

Lynch, Ch. 18, Bereavement issues and spirituality, 242-256

Recommended Readings

Mann & Tarantola, Ch. 29 Are we learning from the lessons of the past?, 302-209

Session 15   FINAL PAPER

University of Chicago
School of Social Service Administration
Chicago, IL

Course Title: Gender and Chronic Health Conditions: Problems and Issues (SSA 444)
Spring Quarter 1997

Course Instructor: Laura Pankow

DESCRIPTION

Health care accounts for a disproportionate amount of the gross national product (GNP) absorbed in the United States. Health care is an industry that does not follow the economic rules of supply and demand. As use increases, so does cost. Reasons for the increasing cost of health care are: (1) the "baby boomer" generation is aging and older people are more likely than other parts of the population to develop chronic health conditions requiring consistent and expensive medical treatment, (2) modern medical technology is expensive, and (3) many people use medical services when these services are not necessary. Health psychology is a field employing the expertise of many disciplines which operates within the medical system and outside of it. Health and human behavior addresses issues beyond psychological processes (i.e., adapting to life with a chronic health condition), which exist as a result of the connection between mental health and medicine. Health psychology also includes topics beyond the individual. Human response to health problems is determined by many factors and is best studied from multiple positions.

This course will be conducted as a seminar. Readings, lectures, and discussions will include material from many disciplines. The definition of health by the World Health Organization—"a complete state of physical, mental, and social well being and not merely the absence of disease or infirmity"— will serve as our guide for a holistic approach to the study of gender and response to chronic health problems.

Because the course will specifically address the influence of gender on incidence, approach to treatment, and research in the areas of health and behavior, issues of diversity and social work values/ethics are inherent topics discussed in this course (see specifically M6.5.1–M6.6 of the CSWE Curriculum Policy Statement).

OBJECTIVES

Upon completing this course students will be able to:

*   identify societal misconceptions regarding chronic health conditions such as diabetes mellitus and arthritis

*   recognize the need to varying approaches to intervention with clients with chronic health conditions based on gender

*   be cognizant of the fact that conclusions drawn from epidemiological statistics are not transferable to an individual

- recognize and employ the need for multifaceted perspectives on health and human behavior
- have a better understanding of the provisions of the Americans with Disabilities Act and have knowledge of resources from which to obtain information about equipping a business for a disabled employee

TEXTS

Kaplan, R., Sallis, J., & Patterson, T. (1993). *Health and human behavior.* New York: McGraw-Hill. Reading packet can be purchased in the SSA Production Room.

REQUIREMENTS

1. Students are expected to attend class, have done the assigned reading, and be prepared to participate in class discussions.

2. Students will be expected to write and turn in for evaluation four papers during the quarter that integrate the readings.
   - There are 10 units in this course. Students will select four units upon which to submit papers.
   - The paper for each unit will be due at the beginning of the class period following the presentation/discussion of that unit.
   - The MAXIMUM length of these papers is to be four double-spaced, typed pages. Use Courier 10 cpi type font (or its equivalent) and margins of no smaller than one inch top and bottom and left and right. Papers not meeting these specifications are not acceptable and will not be graded.
   - These papers are not to be summaries of the readings. "Integration" means that you have read the material, pondered it and considered the strengths and weaknesses of the studies. You should identify unanswered questions. Read with a critical eye, then discuss ways in which these questions could be addressed. Keep research methods in mind. Your "ways" of solving problems should offer improvements over the studies you've read, not contribute to further demise!

3. An oral presentation of 20–30 minutes will be required of each student.
   - Each student must pick a unique topic for the presentation.
   - Gender and other diversity issues should be a focal point of your presentation. How do gender and other aspects of diversity affect the chronic health condition that you are presenting?
   - Any topic may be selected from the following list. These are broad topics so talk to me about a specific aspect that you want to present and I will be able to help you with resources. You may also select a topic not included in the list as long as it is approved by the instructor prior to the presentation.
   - Dependent upon the number of students in the class, we will have 1-2 presentations per class session. Pick a topic as soon as possible, as presentation dates will be given on a first come/ first serve basis.

List of Topics

chronic pain	head injury	smoking
arthritis	violence	obesity
diabetes mellitus	substance abuse	dementia
cardiovascular disease	dietary risk factors and intervention	sickle cell disease/trait
cancer		osteoporosis
AIDS	physical activity	

GRADING
Grades will be based on three factors: Class participation in discussion, 20%; Synthesis Papers, 40%; Class Presentation: 40%

OUTLINE
(See Bibliography for complete references to packet readings)

Week 1
Introduction to course and discussion of syllabus/course requirements
Introduction to Health Psychology

Readings:
Text (Kaplan et al.): Chapter 1

Reading Packet
Reddy, Fleming, & Adesso (1992). Gender and health.
Leviton (1996). Integrating psychology and public health.

Week 2
Health behavior and epidemiology

Readings
Text (Kaplan et al.): Chapter 2

Reading Packet
Anderson (1995). Behavioral and sociocultural perspectives on ethnicity and health.
Schoenborn (1991). The Alameda study—25 years later.

Week 3
Acquired Immune Deficiency Syndrome (AIDS)

Readings
Text (Kaplan et al.): Chapter 12

Reading Packet
Chesney (1993). Health psychology in the 21st century.
Thode (1997). AIDS does not discriminate against gays—or anyone else.

In-class video: Womansource HIV (Burroughs Wellcome Company)

Week 4
Sickle Cell Anemia

Reading Packet
Pankow (1996). Race and motivation toward parenthood.
Samuels-Reid et al. (1984). Contraceptive practices and reproductive patterns in sickle cell disease.
Neal-Cooper & Scott (1988). Genetic counseling in sickle cell anemia.

Week 5
Arthritis and Pain

Readings
Text (Kaplan et al.): Chapter 8

Reading Packet
Park (1994). Self-regulation and control of rheumatic disorders.
Dunbar-Jacob (1993). Contributions to patient adherence.

Week 6
Cardiovascular Disease

Readings
Text (Kaplan et al.): Chapter 10

Reading Packet
Barefoot et al. (1981). Hostility, CHD incidence, and total mortality.
Kaplan et al. (1992). Does lowering cholesterol cause increases in depression, suicide, and accidents?

Week 7
Diabetes Mellitus

Readings
Text (Kaplan et al.): Chapter 9

Reading Packet
Johnson (1993). Compliance and control in insulin-dependent diabetics.
Barron (1978). Blindness and diabetes from a psychologist's perspective.

Week 8
Visual Impairment

Reading Packet

Pankow (1992). Seeing through the patient's eyes.

Pankow (1995). Comparison of locus of control among nursing home residents with visual impairment and normal sight.

Pankow, Pliskin, & Luchins (1996). An optical intervention for visual hallucinations associated with visual impairment and dementia in the elderly.

Week 9

Disorders Associated with Reproductive Changes with Aging

Reading Packet

Friedman & Weinberg (1995). Breast cancer screening behaviors and intentions among asymptomatic women 50 years of age and older.

Hampton (1991). Reproductive system: Changes in reproductive physiology.

Week 10

Americans with Disabilities Act

Reading Packet

U.S. Equal Employment Opportunity Commission. (1992). Title I (An overview of legal requirements), Title II (Who is protected by the ADA?), and Title III (The reasonable accommodation obligation).

BIBLIOGRAPHY

Anderson, N. (1995). Behavioral and sociocultural perspectives on ethnicity and health. *Health Psychology, 14,* 649-653.

Barefoot, M., Dahlstrom, W., & Willias, R. (1981). Hostility, CHD incidence, and total mortality: A 25 year follow-up study of 255 physicians. *Przeglad Psychologicz, 27,* 705-711.

Barron, S. (1978). Blindness and diabetes from a psychologist's perspective. *Journal of Visual Impairment and Blindness, 72,* 354-357.

Burroughs Wellcome Company. (1993). *Womansource HIV.* (Video)

Chesney, M. (1993). Health psychology in the 21st century: Acquired immune deficiency syndrome as a harbinger of things to come. *Health Psychology, 12,* 259-268.

DiMatteo, M., Sherbourne, C., Hays, R., Ordway, L., Kravitz, R., McGlynn, E., Kaplan, S., & Rogers, W. (1993). Physicians' characteristics influence patients' adherence to medical treatment: Results from the medical outcomes study. *Health Psychology, 12,* 93-102.

Dunbar-Jacob, J. (1993). Contributions to patient adherence: Is it time to share the blame? *Health Psychology, 12,* 91-92.

Equal Employment Opportunity Commission. (1992). *A technical assistance manual on the employment provisions (Title I) of the Americans with Disabilities Act.* Washington, DC: Author.

Friedman, L., & Weinberg, A. (1995). Breast cancer screening behaviors and intentions among asymptomatic women 50 years of age and older. *American Journal of Preventive Medicine, 11,* 218-223.

Hampton, J. (1991). Reproductive system: Changes in reproductive physiology. In J. Hampton (Ed.), *The Biology of Human Aging*. Dubuque, IA: William C. Brown.

Johnson, S. (1993). Compliance and control in insulin dependent diabetes: Does behavior really make a difference? In N. Schneiderman & P. McCabe (Eds.), *Perspectives in Behavioral Medicine* (pp. 275-297). Hillsdale, NJ: Lawrence Erlbaum.

Kaplan, R., Manuch, S., & Shumaker, S. (1992). Does lowering cholesterol cause increases in depression, suicide, and accidents? In H. Friedman, et al. (Eds.), *Hostility, Coping, and Health* (pp. 47-123. Washington, DC: American Psychological Association.

Kaplan, R., Sallis, J., & Patterson, T. (1993). *Health and Human Behavior*. New York: McGraw-Hill.

Leviton, L. (1996, Jan.). Integrating psychology and public health: Challenges and opportunities. *American Psychologist*, 42-51.

Neal-Cooper, F., & Scott, R. (1988). Genetic counseling in sickle cell anemia: Experience with couples at risk. *Public Health Reports, 103*, 174-178.

Pankow, L. (1992). Seeing through the patient's eyes. *Journal of the American Optometric Association, 63*, 678-679.

Pankow, L. (1995). Comparison of locus of control among nursing home residents with visual impairment and normal sight. *Journal of the American Optometric Association, 66*, 613-619.

Pankow, L., Pliskin, N., & Luchins, D. (1996). An optical intervention for visual hallucinations associated with visual impairment and dementia in elderly patients. *Journal of Neuropsychiatry and Clinical Neurosciences, 8*, 88-92.

Pankow, L. (1996). *Race and motivation toward parenthood: Implications for genetic counseling addressing family planning and sickle cell disease/trait*. Unpublished manuscript.

Park, D. (1994). Self-regulation and control of rheumatic disorders. In S. Maes, H. Leventhal, & M. Johnson (Eds.), *International Review of Health Psychology* (Vol. 3) (pp. 189-217). New York: Wiley.

Reddy, D., Fleming, R., & Adesso, V. (1992). In S. Maes, H. Leventhal, & M. Johnson (Eds.), *International Review of Health Psychology* (pp. 3-32). New York: Wiley.

Samuels-Reid, J., Scott, R., & Brown, W. (1984). Contraceptive practices and reproductive patterns in sickle cell disease. *Journal of the National Medical Association, 76*, 879-883.

Schoenborn, C. (1991). The Alameda study: 25 years later. In S. Maes, H. Leventhal, & M. Johnson (Eds.), *International Review of Health Psychology* (Vol. 2) (pp. 80-116). New York: Wiley.

Thode, J. (1997, Feb. 19). AIDS does not discriminate against gays—or anyone else. *South Bend Tribune*, p. A-7.

University of Chicago
School of Social Service Administration,
Harris Graduate School of Public Policy Studies, and
Pritzker School of Medicine
Chicago, IL

Course Title: Health Care for the Poor (SSA 486, Medicine 604, Pediatrics 469, Public Policy 478)
Spring 1997

Course Instructor: Deborah Burnet

INTRODUCTION

"Health Care Delivery to the Poor" is a classroom course offered each spring. It is attended by students from medicine, social services, public policy, and law schools. Students learn about provision of health care services for the poor and barriers to effective delivery of care. Each year current issues in health care policy and reform efforts are reviewed. Site visits to Cook County Hospital and other clinical settings are an important component of this class.

Other classroom offerings include courses in domestic violence and health care policy and ethics. Students and housestaff interested in health care for the poor can find a variety of offerings at the University of Chicago, and many faculty members will be available to support their efforts in pursuing these interests.

DESCRIPTION

In this course, we explore issues related to health care delivery for the poor. Each year we focus on a certain topic current in health care policy for several of the class sessions. This year we will focus on Medicaid reform efforts and, in particular, on Medicaid Managed Care. We will review the history and design of Medicaid, study recent changes and directions in the Medicaid program, and try to assess whether Medicaid Managed Care will benefit the poor. We will also take a closer look at several patient populations at special risk.

Most class sessions will be in large-group, lecture/seminar format, many with guest speakers who have experience serving the poor. For some class sessions we will break into two groups for smaller discussion sections. This format will allow students to share their reactions to readings, site visits, and previous speaker presentations. Students will be assigned to one of the two discussion groups. Discussion sections will be led by the teaching assistants.

Students will be expected to do assigned reading, attend classes and discussion sections, and visit Cook County Hospital and at least one community health center. Information and schedules for site visits will be forthcoming. Three brief (1- to 2-page) reaction papers are expected in response to your two site visits and to one of the readings. These are not research papers; they are simply your thoughts and reactions to the reading or the site visit experience. For 100 credits, students will also write a final paper (approx. 8–10 pages). Two or three topics relevant to class work will be suggested; however, other topics pertinent to health care for the poor may be considered. Final paper topics are due in the fifth week of class; final papers are due the eighth week. Students may choose to work collaboratively in groups of two or three to produce a longer paper if desired.

READING LIST

William Julius Wilson, *The Truly Disadvantaged: The Inner City, the Underclass, and Public Policy.* Chicago: University of Chicago Press, 1987.

Laurie Kaye Abraham, *Mama Might Be Better off Dead: The Failure of Urban Health Care in America.* Chicago: University of Chicago Press, 1993.

Abraham Verghese, *My Own Country: A Doctor's Story of a Town and Its People in the Age of AIDS.* New York: Simon and Schuster, 1994.

Additional articles will be assigned for several class sessions.

CLASS SCHEDULE

Weeks 1–3 Health Care Delivery in the United States
Session 1a   Class intro; Introduction to U.S. Health Care Delivery System
                Deborah Burnet, M.D.

Session 1b   Private Health Insurance: Who's In and Who's Out?
                Hank Webber, University of Chicago Vice President for Administration

Session 2a   Health Care Financing in the United States
                Ed Lawlor, School of Public Policy

Session 2b   Ethics of Caring for the Poor
                John Lantos, Center for Clinical Medical Ethics

Session 3a   Medicaid
                Art Kohrmann, Children's Memorial Hospital

Session 3b   Managed Care — Will it Work for the Poor? Panel Discussion:
                Quentin Young, M.D., and Bob Burger, Illinois Associations of HMOs

Weeks 4–9 Groups at Special Risk
Session 4a   The African-American "Underclass"
                Barak Obama, Illinois State Senator

Session 4b   Small-Group Discussions — William Julius Wilson, *The Truly Disadvantaged* (Chapters 1, 2, 5, 7)

Session 5a   FINAL PAPER TOPICS DUE
              The Physically and Developmentally Disabled
              Jim Fruehling, Bethphage Mission, Inc.

Session 5b   Women at Risk—Domestic Violence
              Dawn Emmons Julian, Loop YWCA

Session 6a   Long-Term Care and the Elderly
              Marc Paloma, UCH Social Services

Session 6b   Small-Group Discussions—Laurie Kaye Abraham, *Mama Might Be Better Off Dead*

Session 7a   HIV/AIDS
              Neel French, Weiss Memorial Hospital

Session 7b   Discussion Groups—Abraham Verghese, *My Own Country*

Session 8a   Final Papers Due
              Small-Group Discussion—Cook County Hospital Visit Reactions

Session 8b   Men and "Others" Who Fall through the Cracks—The County System as Safety Net
              Ruth Rothstein, Cook County Hospital

Session 9a   Children and Adolescents
              Nancy Fritz, Austin School-Based Clinic

Session 9b   Violence as a Public Health Issue
              Sue Avila, Cook County Trauma Unit

Week 10 — Putting it All Together
Session 10a   Realistic Options for Health Care Reform in the United States

Session 10b   Discussion Groups—Health Care for the Poor; Where Do We Go from
              Here?

APPENDIX
Opportunities for Students and Residents

Students and housestaff who are interested in health care for the poor can choose from several offerings when they have elective time. Clinical opportunities include rotations at the New City Health Center, Lawndale Christian Health Center, Woodlawn Maternal and Child Health Center, and other sites. Several classroom courses open to medical students and those from other disciplines also explore topics related to health care for the poor.

- New City Health Center is a community-based clinic located in an indigent area about four miles west of the university. Services include pediatrics, internal medicine, obstetrics and gynecology, and family practice. Some University of Chicago faculty members see patients there on a part-time basis, and the clinic has eight full-time physicians, as well. Students and residents can choose to rotate there for a month at a time, or they can arrange a long-term continuity experience, seeing patients once or twice a week for several months. Preceptor sessions held concurrently with the clinical experience seek to address the impact of social circumstances upon health.

- Lawndale Christian Health Center is located on Chicago's West Side. It also provides a variety of health services to community residents in an indigent area. The clinic is part of a spectrum of services offered by the Lawndale Community Church, which also addresses community needs in the areas of housing, hunger, etc. The clinic is church-based, in that most of its staff are members of the church there and see their health professions as an extension of their religious commitment. This rotation is available to senior students on either a monthly basis or once a week for a longer term.

- Woodlawn Maternal and Child Health Center is located right across the midway from the university (a 10-minute walk). It serves residents of the low-income neighborhood just south of the university. Health services are provided to women and children, including prenatal and gynecological care, pediatrics, teen clinic, and family planning services. Pediatrics residents rotate there on a regular basis, and elective time is available to interested students as well. Services may expand to include internal medicine in the future.

Students and housestaff can also set up electives at clinical sites of their own choosing. A faculty member will be available to act as a preceptor for these ventures. In the past, students and residents have rotated at various community clinics throughout Chicago, at Indian Health Service facilities around the country, and abroad in various Third World settings.

Appendix

COUNCIL ON SOCIAL WORK EDUCATION
Publications and Media Commission

Instrument for Evaluating Course Outlines

Please ensure that the syllabi you solicit and send to the Council for publication are evaluated using criteria similar to the following.

1. Descriptiveness and accuracy of course title.

Exemplary	Very Good	Good	Fair	Poor
+_____	+_____	+_____	+_____	+

2. Comprehensiveness of content (given focus and length of course).

Exemplary	Very Good	Good	Fair	Poor
+_____	+_____	+_____	+_____	+

3. Range of perspectives represented within topic area.

Exemplary	Very Good	Good	Fair	Poor
+_____	+_____	+_____	+_____	+

4. Relevance of course content to social work.

Exemplary	Very Good	Good	Fair	Poor
+_____	+_____	+_____	+_____	+

5. Currency of course content and readings.

Exemplary	Very Good	Good	Fair	Poor
+_____	+_____	+_____	+_____	+

6. Creativity and innovation (e.g., in assignments and instruction).

Exemplary	Very Good	Good	Fair	Poor
+_____	+_____	+_____	+_____	+

7. Organization of course content.

Exemplary	Very Good	Good	Fair	Poor
+_____	+_____	+_____	+_____	+

8. Clarity of course outline.

Exemplary	Very Good	Good	Fair	Poor
+_____	+_____	+_____	+_____	+

9. Inclusion of content on special populations, as required by the Curriculum Policy Statement.

Exemplary	Very Good	Good	Fair	Poor
+_____	+_____	+_____	+_____	+

10. Clarity of student assessment procedures.

Exemplary	Very Good	Good	Fair	Poor
+_____	+_____	+_____	+_____	+

11. Potential use by faculty in other social work programs.

Exemplary	Very Good	Good	Fair	Poor
+_____	+_____	+_____	+_____	+